# MODERN AILMENTS

# ANCIENT REMEDIES

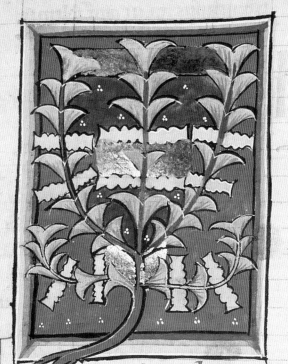

upales: epanthenon. Egypti: ũ.
otetijm. Itali: crocatim Quidama͛te
latiridem eam appellant. Vna
cura eǐ: ad durtiem stomachi.
herbam latiridis granium cum
poptime purgatum fuit.
inaqua calida potatum dabis. sta
tim alueum purgat̃: reum sanat.
Nomen huiuf herbe lactuca lepo
rina dr̃.

Er aute meadem. Item. ○○○
herba umbilico infantium dͥ
ta rimposita pfectissime mede͛r
ipsanat. Nomen ustuf herbe lati
rdis nuncupatur.

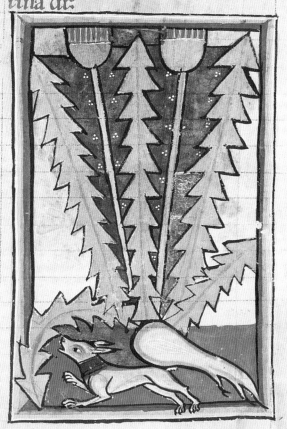

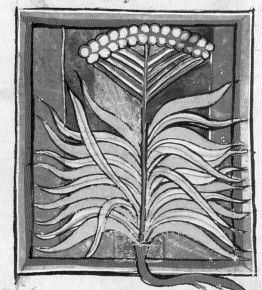

A grecis siquidem dr̃ cocosindos.
Quidam ũ camellam eam uocãt.

Nascitur in locis cultis rsablosis.
lep̃ autem inestate cum animo de
ficit. hanc herbam comedit. ideoq;
lactuca leporina dicĩ. Prima cu
ra ipsius. ad remediandum feb
herbam lactucam lecttantem:

# MODERN AILMENTS

# ANCIENT REMEDIES

*a healing manual*

GILLIAN KERR N.D. AND DR. YVONNE BLOOMFIELD

SMITHMARK

# CONTENTS

## INTRODUCTION 6
• The many properties of herbs
• The herbal wisdom of ancient physicians
• The basics of looking after ourselves

## OTHER ANCIENT REMEDIES FOR MODERN AILMENTS 82

• Food and nutrition • Aromatherapy
• Traditional Chinese medicine • Massage
• Cleansing techniques • Yoga
• Practical home remedies

## A–Z OF MODERN AILMENTS

# INTRODUCTION

Modern medicine has made huge changes in the way we view and manage our day-to-day upsets and illnesses. Recently, however, many people have decided that we may be paying too high a price — in terms of side effects, after-effects, and related stress effects — with our widespread use of new, technologically enhanced chemical drugs. It seems that many of us have decided that it's time to regain control of our lives, our health and our future.

Taking control of our health requires a fair bit of work, at least to start with. Most of us have become so busy that we seldom make time to look after ourselves. It's quicker, easier, more convenient and sometimes even cheaper — in terms of time lost from work — to pop in to the doctor or pharmacist for a quick-cure prescription. But at what cost?

Are there more "modern ailments," or is today's fast-track lifestyle creating them? Have we swapped the plague for AIDS, debility for chronic fatigue syndrome, ague for modern-day allergies? Could it be that somewhere along the way, with the help of technology and exciting chemical advances, we might have changed the nature of many germs, viruses, bacteria and infections? Have we let loose a stream of synthetic pharmaceuticals that have resulted in these infectious agents mutating into more virulent little critters?

Perhaps it is time for us to join the worldwide trend of people embracing both the best of the old tried-and-true herbal traditions and the expertise of modern medicine in order to live happier, healthier and more productive lives.

### THE MANY PROPERTIES OF HERBS

Increasingly, we are turning back to ancient ways and making use of Nature's natural pharmacy, with its huge, potent, unpretentious and widely proven medicine-chest filled with herbs.

The word "herb" comes from the Sanskrit word "to eat," which later became the Latin word *herba*, meaning grass or fodder. A herb is defined botanically as a plant with a fleshy rather than woody stem that, after blooming, dies down to the ground. As it happens, there are a few herbs with woody stems, such as sage, thyme and rosemary, but there are exceptions in nature just as there are in human nature.

An herb has properties that enable us to use it as as food or medicine, or for its scent or flavor. Many of the herbs we use today as seasonings were originally used as medicines. Turmeric is a good example. Most people treat it merely as "poor man's saffron" and use it to color their rice. Yet in India, turmeric is used as widely as a medicinal home remedy to treat bruising, inflammation and infections — as aspirin is used in the West.

Throughout the world, from earliest times, herbs have been used for a multitude of purposes. They have been used in foods, drinks, medicines, poisons, cosmetics, incenses and even clothing, fibers and paper.

Our distant ancestors were hunter-gatherers who used all sorts of plants in their daily lives. Over time they determined which ones were bitter or poisonous; which ones were nourishing or soothing; which ones could be used for foods or medicine; and which ones provided mind-altering effects when brewed, inhaled or ingested. They gained their knowledge through a process of live and learn — which is what we are still doing today.

Throughout history, herbs have been used for magical purposes, to create love or death potions, for divination and in religious and state ceremonies. Herbs were considered powerful and had an important role in the rituals that enhanced traditional life. Herbs could make or break dynasties: the Borgias, for example, rid themselves of unwanted family, friends and foes with pledges made in poisoned herbal wines.

## THE HERBAL WISDOM OF ANCIENT PHYSICIANS

The ancient Egyptians believed that the heart was the source of 36 channels to the rest of the body and that blockages in these channels caused sickness. They believed that pain was caused by substances that entered the body from outside and could be countered by the use of special protective herbs. Their herbal treatments (such as the use of rotten bread for infection) and early surgical procedures (such as the use of flour and water to make a cast for a broken limb) were ridiculed in more recent

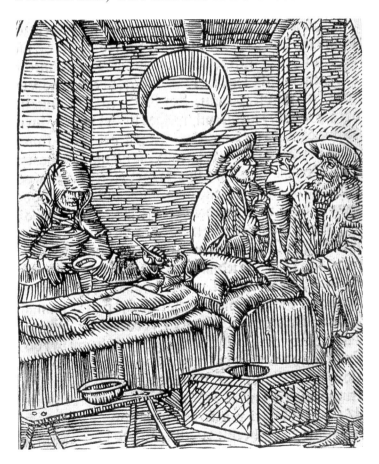

times, until modern science showed why these treatments worked. We now know that, among many things, the ancient Egyptians knew the effectiveness of penicillin and plaster casts.

Ancient Egyptian physicians were renowned for their skills. In fact, one of their doctors became so famous that he was later revered as a god — Imhotep, the god of Healing.

The Ayurvedic medical discipline developed in India from approximately 3000 B.C. and is still widely practiced today. Ayurvedic physicians concern themselves with the functioning of body and spirit as a whole, rather than focusing on a single organ or disease symptom. Their use of herbal medicines has come down through the centuries to provide the backbone of India's modern medicine practices.

Ancient Sumerian records, dating back to 3000 B.C., refer widely to the medicinal actions of many herbs that are still widely used, and the first recorded Chinese herbal text, written around 2700 B.C., lists more than 300 herbs and their actions and therapeutic effects.

Traditional Chinese medicine is the complex and fascinating system in which herbs are used extensively. A balancing of the two fundamental principles of Chinese philosophy — yin, the feminine, passive, dark, cold principle; and yang, the masculine, active, light, hot principle — is the cornerstone of this system. The Chinese physician takes everything about the patient into account. The patient's background, genetic history, present symptoms, psychological state, diet and lifestyle are all appraised and considered in relation to the nature of the disease and its progress. Following diagnosis, a combination of herbs and treatment are brought together to balance the yin/yang energy in the body, thus creating health and harmony of mind, body and spirit.

The Chinese believe that "the superior physician treats the patient before the illness is manifested. It is only the inferior physician who treats the illness he was unable to prevent."

The ancient Greeks and Romans used herbs for many purposes. Dioscorides' treatise on medicinal herbs, written in the first century, remained an authoritative reference for the western world well into the seventeenth century. The Greeks' god of healing, Aesculapius, the son of Apollo, is symbolized by the serpent entwined around a staff, which is today the symbol of the medical practitioner.

It was probably in Aristotle's time, in the fourth century B.C., that traditional medicine and early pharmaceutical medicine began to diverge. At this time, the role of the physician became acknowledged as legitimate, and the role of the entrepreneurial "drug" marketers began to expand. But the ancient concept — look to the individual, treat the person, not just the symptom — and in fact, all traditional medicines have a great deal in common with the classical Greek approach. These are generally rooted in a holistic view of health care.

Traditional medicine has many forms, some formal and regularized, others informal and undocumented. While most of the oldest forms are mainly folkloric, magical and religious in nature, some of the more developed ancient forms, such as those found in India and China, were comparable to Western medicine, prior to the scientific revolution of the last two hundred years, in their organization and application. Ancient texts provided the framework, and modern holistic medicine is still based on the wisdom from these writings.

The fifteenth, sixteenth and seventeenth centuries proved to be the "Golden Age" for European and British herbals, as information became available in local languages, rather than only in Latin or Greek. The most famous scientist and researcher in the seventeenth century was probably the Englishman Nicholas Culpepper (1616–54), whose unique mixture of traditional medicine, research, folklore and magic provided many remedies for the common folk. Culpepper started as a humble apothecary who went on to write the *English Physician* in 1651. These remedies, easily made from common ingredients, were used widely as treatments for the many medical complaints faced by an increasingly urbanized population. Other great herbals were written by John Gerard (in 1597) and Parkinson (in 1640).

In the eighteenth and nineteenth centuries there were great developments in surgery, chemistry, biochemistry and pharmacy. A new industry began, engineering scientifically developed drugs based on the chemical formulas of herbs. These drugs provided an easy alternative to having to "do it yourself" at

a time when increasing numbers of people were taking on factory work and were thus unable to grow herbs or find the time for preparing medicines at home. It was during this period that the use of herbal medicines went into decline and the pharmaceutical industry began to establish its power base.

Attitudinal shifts have also played a part in the change. In 1948 the Public Health Act was introduced in Britain, enabling everyone to obtain free medical treatment. This led to a change in people's attitudes — and they came to believe that responsibility for their health and well-being lay with the government rather than with themselves; this has become a common attitude in many parts of the Western world.

Another belief that has become increasingly evident in the West as the twentieth century has progressed is the belief that modern pharmaceutical drugs are cure-alls, and that there is no longer any need to take care of the "self." If we become ill, we can simply take a course of pills and be cured.

To a large extent, twentieth-century Westerners have thrown out the wisdom handed down by earlier generations. There hasn't been the time, or the need, to bother with herbal medicines. But attitudes are now changing and we are starting to see that balance is probably the key.

People are discovering the benefits of combining the best of the old traditions with the expertise of the new. In the modern Western world, where our energies are being consumed in the pursuit of material success at the cost of contentment and harmony, we are constantly seeking new ways to achieve some sort of balance and consistency of energy. While we no longer need to fear scurvy, typhoid, smallpox, epidemics and plagues, we now face cancer, AIDS, chronic fatigue syndrome and a variety of stressful new allergies and other modern-day afflictions. And there are still many ailments which cannot be fixed through the use of modern pharmaceutical drugs.

In much of the world, immunization has had a major impact on health, freeing millions from the scourge of many killer diseases. But are some of us suffering side effects from taking vaccines? That's a big question confronting the medical world. Many naturopathic schools of thought believe we have changed one set of ills for another, and a growing number of people are turning to the "back to nature" approach, rather than the "fix it quick and forget the consequences" attitude which has become so widespread.

### THE BASICS OF LOOKING AFTER OURSELVES

The ancients, and good old Mother Nature, have shown us time and again that the body will heal itself, given the right conditions. There are plenty of choices to be had in this world and a wide variety of authorities to tell us how to make them, but ultimately your healing is up to you. This book aims to clarify the choices that are available.

Health is about being alive in your self, and being happy with your self. The best medicine is the one that works for you, and becoming informed is the first step in your healing process and your self-empowerment. All the herbal remedies covered here are simple, and in most cases they've stood the test of thousands of years of time.

Read as much as you can about the various herbs and their uses and about any conditions that affect you or your family, then talk it over with professionals whom you respect and can communicate with openly. You will then be in a position to make informed decisions as to how you wish to manage the healing process. Think about the way you would like things to happen and try to visualize your perfect scenario. You'll be surprised how solutions can come to you when you stop trying to force issues by just allowing things to evolve.

All the herbal treatments and remedies provided here can help you reduce stress and enhance your sense of well-being without the side effects of the modern pharmaceutical drugs.

Many of the old traditions have much to offer us. Take the notion of convalescence. In the old days, after sickness, there was a period of time called convalescence when you were given space and support to recover. Today, when time is money, you are expected to return to work immediately following an illness. In fact, most of us tend to feel guilty about being away from work at all. So we don't give ourselves time to regain vitality, and our immune system struggles along till the next time, when it breaks down again because it just can't cope.

The simple rules still apply: when the body needs to rest, let it. A tired body is probably telling you you're out of balance. Take time to relax. Stop, look and listen. Remember there's another world out there — one that's just a moment away from where you are now. If you take time to get into a different "space" you'll be able to come back to the here and now with a clearer perspective. It's your life.

Rest is a simple, wonderful healing remedy, yet most of us "soldier on" when we have colds, headaches or the flu, feeling we must go to work and perform. Failing to listen to a tired body's calls for help — often the need for the simplest remedies and rest — will result in working yourself into the ground. And for what? Material goods you're too tired or unwell to enjoy? Alienated families? Burned-out body, mental tension, anxiety and stress as your daily companions?

Sleep is also vital to your health. It is essential for restoring energy and optimism and allowing the body to rebuild its reserves. If you don't sleep well for one night, it's annoying; but if you lose the ability to sleep well at all you will seriously deplete your body's reserves. The Chinese would say you are starting to erode your essential chi, your life-force energy, leaving you open to all sorts of infections which a healthy immune system could zap in a flash.

If you've begun a pattern of sleepless nights and stressful days, consider using some of nature's gentle assistants, such as chamomile, valerian and some of the other helper herbs you can read about in this book.

Stress has come to play a huge part in our lives and we need to look at how we can deal with it. Here are some guidelines:

• Take time out.
• Find your own center.
• Stop, look, listen and learn.
• Learn from ancient wisdom, and then create your own.
• Best of all, try a few of the herbal helpers growing right outside your back door. You won't need a script.

From ancient times, herbs have helped all sorts of people with all sorts of conditions in all sorts of cultures. Ancient remedies can lead to modern cures.

When using this book, check out the herbal section to see how you can stay healthy using preventative measures, and cross reference these with the section covering modern ailments. If you're in any doubt though, see your medical practitioner or qualified naturopath before you make any life-changing decisions. The aim is for us to be healthy, happy and well-balanced. Remember, it's up to you.

# A-Z

## OF HERBAL REMEDIES

# ALFALFA

Lucerne, buffalo herb, purple medic
*Medicago sativa*
**FAMILY:** Papilionaceae

*Alfalfa is the great alkalizer. It has been a time-honored organic contributor to soil, enhancing its structure and mineral content throughout the ages. Alfalfa is a powerful nutritive tonic and counteracts bodily disorders caused by excessive acid.*

**DESCRIPTION:** The erect, smooth stem grows from an elongated deep tap root to a height of 12–18 inches (30–45 cm), and bears succulent green leaves. Its clover-like spikes of blue or purplish flowers grow from June to August in the northern hemisphere, finally producing the characteristic spirally coiled seed pods. Alfalfa is a perennial, although it may require three to four years' cultivation until attaining full growth.

*Alfalfa is a hormone-like and alkalizing herb that helps to balance blood calcium levels. It has estrogen-mimicking properties and contains fat-splitting enzymes which can assist in weight control.*

**HISTORY:** The name *Medicago* is derived from Medea in North Africa where this important and ancient plant, widely used medicinally by the Greeks, is thought to have originated. It was not known in northwestern Europe until the seventeenth century when it was given the name *lucerna*, meaning lamp, after the bright, shiny appearance of the seeds. Alfalfa has been used for centuries to sweeten pastures depleted of minerals by overuse. When in cultivation, plant members of this family add nitrogen to the soil via nodules on the roots. For centuries, alfalfa has provided a rich source of organic minerals for ensuing crops, when dug back into the soil.

**MODERN USES:** Alfalfa is useful for alkalizing the system, relieving gastritis, stomach ulcers, nausea, cystitis and bladder irritations. It is rich in vitamins A, B2, B6, C, D and K, and contains eight essential amino acids and eight essential digestive enzymes. If taken every day, it is a tonic herb that can enhance the appetite.

Alfalfa is also a hormone-like herb. It has estrogenic properties and may help increase the flow of breast milk. With its natural iodine, it affects the parathyroid glands whose hormones act on the stabilization of calcium in serum blood levels, possibly assisting period pain and premenstrual syndrome. Alfalfa contains fat-splitting enzymes as well, and is often used for weight control.

Rheumatism, sciatica and arthritis can be treated with alfalfa as it helps eliminate excess uric acid. It has been shown to assist the normal clotting of blood, so may be useful in some circulatory disorders.

**AVAILABLE FORMS:** Alfalfa can be obtained as herbal extract, infusion, tablets and sprouted seeds. If using it as a tea, combine it with peppermint or caraway. Use the seeds as a decoction.

*alfalfa*

15

# ALOE VERA

Aloe, Barbados aloe, the burn plant
*Aloe vera & other species*
**FAMILY:** Liliaceae

*At least 180 species of aloe have been used for their beauty, medicinal and skin-care properties. Aloe vera, a member of the lily family, is a succulent, resembling a cactus.*

**DESCRIPTION:** A perennial of East and South Africa and the West Indies, aloe is cultivated for its medicinal properties in tropical and sub-tropical regions. The root produces a rosette of fleshy, basal leaves, which are 1–2 feet long (30–60 cm), with spiny margins. The yellow to purplish drooping flower can be 4 feet (120 cm) high. The outside of the leaf is smooth and rubbery to touch, and contains the plant's gelatinous juice.

*Aloe vera's greatest claim is in its success in treating skin conditions. It is invaluable for its immediate, soothing effect on burns, bites and stings. Aloe vera is one of our most versatile herbs.*

**HISTORY:** Cleopatra reputedly used the gel of the aloe vera plant in her bath water and in the colorings for her eyes and lips. Two thousand years ago, the Egyptians called it "The Plant of Immortality." Greek scientists of the same period regarded it as "The Universal Panacea" and the Native Americans named it "The Wand of Heaven." Sixth-century Persians used it as a cathartic, and its name comes from the Arabic word *alloeh* meaning a shining, bitter substance. It has had widespread medicinal and cosmetic use for a variety of conditions — recent scientific research has found more than 70 essential ingredients within the plant, including most vitamins, minerals, enzymes, proteins and amino acids.

**MODERN USES:** Aloe vera is known for its ability to soothe and heal burns, sunburn, scalds, stings, cold sores, sprains, bruises and many skin conditions, by applying the gel to the affected area. It is used for acne, arthritis, fungal diseases such as athlete's foot, scalp problems, hemorrhoids, gum and mouth irritations, ulcers and many other conditions. The juice is said to prevent or draw out infection in wounds. A stabilized dose may be administered internally for conditions such as heartburn, constipation and indigestion; however, if taken internally, a carminative is usually also prescribed, as aloe can have a strong, griping, purgative action and so should be used with caution. Many skin-care, beauty and cosmetic products include aloe as a major ingredient. Research shows that the gel contains a mixture of antibiotic, antiinflammatory and astringent properties, as well as a coagulating agent, pain inhibitor, cell-growth stimulator and scar inhibitor.

**AVAILABLE FORMS:** Aloe vera gel, cream or juice is available at retailers, and extracts of aloe vera are used in some soaps, shampoos, beauty and skin-care products. Growing your own aloe vera and applying its unadulterated gel is easy too.

*aloe vera*

# CALENDULA

Marigold, pot marigold, Mary bud
*Calendula officinalis*
FAMILY: Compositae

*Calendula is a traditional healing agent for the external treatment of wounds, sores and other skin problems, with effective anti-inflammatory and antiseptic properties.*

DESCRIPTION: Calendula is a hardy annual garden plant, growing to a height of 1–2 feet, with a hairy, branching stem. The lower leaves are paddle-shaped, the upper more pointed and stalkless, embracing the stem. It has large, ray-shaped, pale yellow to bright orange terminal flower heads. Its odor is slight and aromatic — and it happily brightens up many window boxes and gardens all over the world.

HISTORY: Originally native to Southern Europe, calendula is now widely cultivated in all temperate climates. Calendula tea has long been used as an ancient remedy for gastritis, ulcers, colitis and diarrhea, and early herbalists recommended it for women with painful menstruation or menopausal problems, and to promote perspiration and to strengthen the heart. Wandering gypsy healers in the seventeenth century advised the regular application of fresh juice to remove warts, and the petals were frequently used in creams and compresses to treat localized skin problems, or made into a gargle for treating mouth ulcers, gingivitis and sore throats. In Tudor times, it was widely used as an antiaging cosmetic and to add golden highlights to the hair; frequently, too, a marigold flower was used to relieve pain and reduce swelling after a bee or wasp sting.

MODERN USES: Calendula is still one of the most popular herbs for stimulating the immune system and preventing infection. It is commonly used in various combinations as a healing and soothing wound lotion or cream. Recent scientific research indicates extract or tincture of calendula significantly stimulates healing and tissue regeneration in wounds. Contributing to the healing antiseptic effect is its proven antibacterial properties.

It is also considered an effective herb of cholagogue activity; that is, it can increase the flow of bile by 20–50 percent. Topically, it is still used as an ingredient in the treatment of varicose veins, hemorrhoids, bruises, sprains and pulled muscles.

An infusion of the flowers can be used for many gastro-intestinal problems, such as ulcers, stomach cramps, colitis, vomiting and diarrhea; for conjunctivitis, insect bites, sunburn, chapped lips, general skin problems and as a facial wash for the complexion.

**AVAILABLE FORMS:** An infusion can be made by adding fresh or dried flower petals to boiling water, steeping and straining, or it may be obtained as an ointment or cream, extract or tincture from most health food shops, pharmacies or naturopathic dispensaries.

*Because of its antiseptic and anti-inflammatory characteristics, calendula is a valuable addition to the medicine cabinet for treating cuts, abrasions, traumatic wounds, bruises and sprains.*

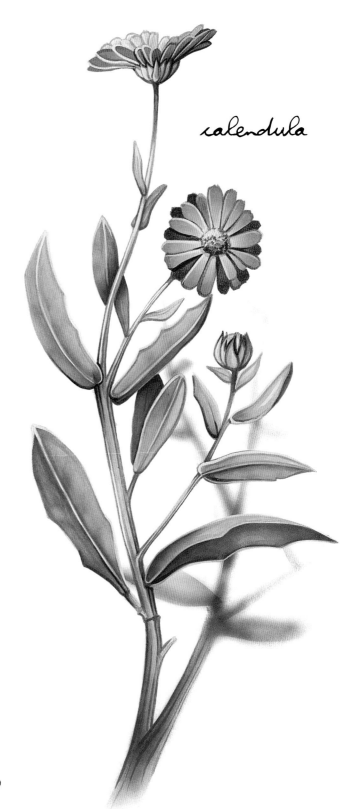

calendula

# CELERY SEED

Garden celery, wild celery, smallage
*Apium graveolens*
**FAMILY:** Umbelliferae

*Celery seeds can provide a foundation for sound nutrition, being high in mineral salts that help remedy diseases such as joint pain or inflexibility while also acting as a tonic for the blood. A keen, active body cleanser.*

**DESCRIPTION:** Celery is a strong-smelling, erect, biennial plant, 1–3 feet (30–90 cm) high, with a fleshy, bulbous root and shiny, dark green pinnate leaves with large, toothed leaflets. The flowers are white or gray white, shortly stalked and often opposite the leaves. There are no upper or lower bracts. The fruit is a small, ribbed elliptical-ovate seed.

**HISTORY:** Celery originated in England and southern Europe, grows in the salty soils of North and South America, Europe and Africa, and is cultivated in other temperate zones. The stalks are used as a food; the seed, medicinally. It has always been used cautiously as a medicine, as it is a strong diuretic and can upset the body's mineral balance. Russian folklore recommended extracting the oil from the root to stimulate sexual potency. An old British remedy for rheumatism was to take one part of honey and one part of goat's cream, and boil; pound a little sulfur with nettles and celery seed, mix with the cream and honey, and apply to the affected area. Indian Ayurvedic physicians used celery seed for colds, flu, hiccups, water retention, poor digestion, arthritis, and liver and spleen ailments.

**MODERN USES:** Celery seed is generally employed as a diuretic, antirheumatic, carminative, nervine, alterative and urinary antiseptic. It is most effective when used for the kidneys, bladder, nervous system, joints and blood. It stimulates kidney function and the excretion of uric acid, and has particular indications for cystitis, rheumatoid arthritis and gout. A decoction of the seeds is beneficial for bronchitis, chest congestion and rheumatism, and the tea can be helpful in clearing up many skin problems or as a stimulating circulatory tonic. Recent research has indicated that celery seed can significantly reduce hypertension. A decoction can be made from the seeds and used for nervousness, depression and apathy. It is combined with other herbs, in particular dandelion root and marshmallow, for its diuretic and demulcent properties, or with alfalfa for arthritic conditions. A reliable dose with which to commence is a teaspoon of the ground or crushed seed to a cup of water daily.

**AVAILABLE FORMS:** Take celery seed as a tea, fresh juice, powder or salt. It is also available in tablet, capsule, tincture or extract form.

*celery seed*

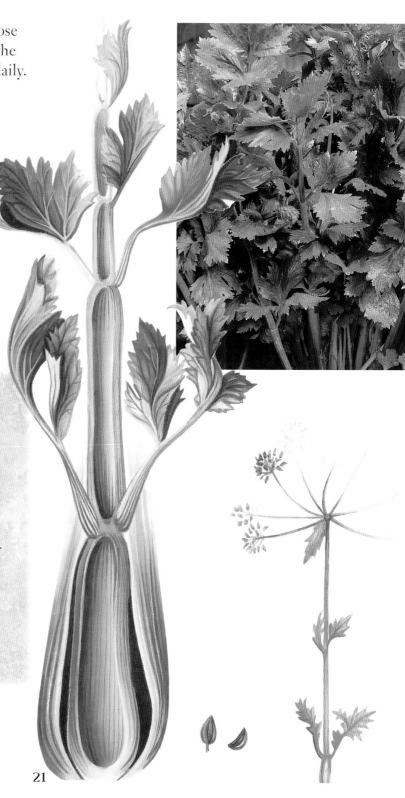

*Celery is a salt-of-the-earth food and medicine which contains a vast array of healing properties, including lowering blood pressure, counteracting body acidity, and relieving the symptoms of arthritis.*

21

# CHAMOMILE

Chamomilla, garden camomile, Roman chamomile
*Anthemis nobilis*
**FAMILY:** Compositae

*Chamomile, such a pretty little plant, and one from that promotes peaceful dreaming —
no wonder it was revered by the Egyptians as a "Herb of the Sun."*

**DESCRIPTION:** The true or common chamomile is a low growing, wispy, creeping annual plant, found wild along roadsides and cultivated in herbal gardens all around the temperate world. It grows easily in chalky or sandy soils, in any sunny position.

Its alternate, downy leaves have 18 or so white-rayed florets, with yellow disk flowers, making them appear quite like a daisy; they are supported on a single erect stalk, drooping when in bud.

*Due to its ease of use, and its gentle action, chamomile is one of the best home remedies for all sorts of modern-day stresses and tensions.*

**HISTORY:** The fresh plant is strongly and pleasantly aromatic with a definite smell of apples, and so it was named by the Greeks "ground-apple" — from *kamai*, meaning on the ground and *melon*, an apple. The Egyptians revered it, and dedicated it to their gods for their belief in its power to cure ague. It was grown for centuries in British country gardens, and known as the "Plant's Physician" for its widespread use as a general domestic medicine for indigestion, stomach troubles and cramps. Interestingly, the Spanish and the Saxons used it for the same reasons, and also named it a sacred herb of the sun.

Many ancient cultures have recorded the many complaints which would benefit from chamomile; in medieval times, it was widely believed to be the only certain remedy for preventing nightmares — this ancient therapeutic use has come down through history to still acknowledge it as a "sleepytime tea."

**MODERN USES:** Chamomile is an anodyne, antispasmodic, carminative, nervine, wound

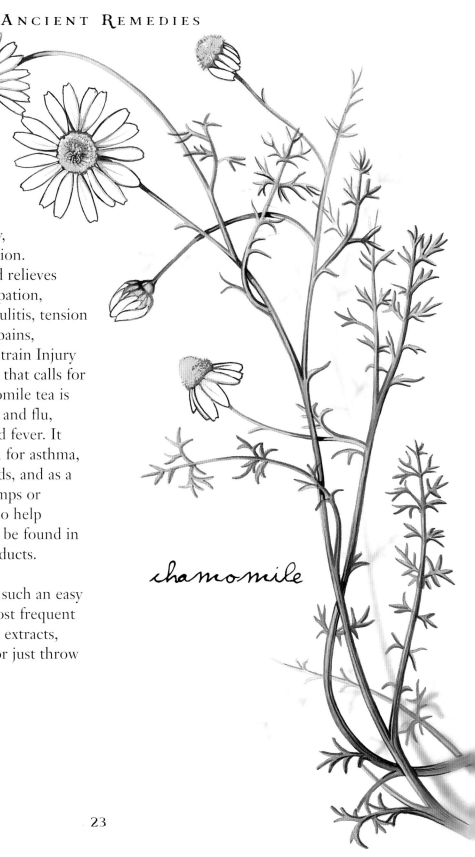

chamomile

healer, uterine relaxant, and tonic that promotes perspiration. It contains the amino acid tryptophan, which acts as a sedative in the body, and is a good source of calcium, magnesium and potassium, the essential phosphates for assisting nervous conditions such as anxiety, restlessness, insomnia and depression. Chamomile improves appetite and relieves indigestion, and is used for constipation, irritable bowel syndrome, diverticulitis, tension headaches, rheumatism and joint pains, muscular tension and Repetitive Strain Injury (RSI) — in fact, for any condition that calls for a calming, soothing effect. Chamomile tea is used for mild stomach ache, colds and flu, teething problems, nightmares and fever. It can also be helpful as a vapor bath for asthma, as a sitz bath to assist hemmorhoids, and as a panacea for painful menstrual cramps or premenstrual syndrome. It will also help blonde hair be blonder, and it can be found in many cosmetics and skin-care products.

**AVAILABLE FORMS:** Chamomile is such an easy and friendly herb to use — the most frequent forms being decoctions, infusions, extracts, oils, teas, tablets and capsules — or just throw a few flowers in the bath to relax.

# DANDELION

Lion's tooth, swine snout, priest's crown
*Taraxacum officinale*
FAMILY: Compositae

*Dandelion is often considered one of the most useful of all herbs, as it has therapeutic properties for the liver, gall bladder, stomach, intestines, kidneys, bladder and blood.*

**DESCRIPTION:** This perennial weed, which grows just about anywhere, is so well known to most people that it hardly needs describing. It has irregular leaves which grow in a rosette from the milky taproot. The root sends up one or more naked flower stems, each terminating in a single yellow flower, which is followed by a cluster of white, parachute-like tufts.

**HISTORY:** Originally native to Western Europe and North Asia, dandelion is now found across the northern temperate zone in pastures, lawns, and along roadsides. The name of the genus comes from the Greek *taraxos*, meaning disorder and *akos*, meaning remedy; the English name derives from the French *dents de lion* referring to its "lion's teeth" leaves.

The herb is rarely mentioned by the ancient Greeks and Romans, but came into widespread use by the Arabs in the eleventh century; by the sixteenth century, it was an official drug in the European pharmacopoeia. The Chinese have known about its antibacterial properties since the seventh century. India's Ayurvedic physicians have used dandelion for over a thousand years for a variety of conditions, including colds, bronchitis, obesity, liver disorders and certain types of ulcers.

**MODERN USES:** The modern herbalist uses dandelion for many conditions, although as in

*With its wide range of therapeutic actions, dandelion forms an important part of many herbal formulas; it is particularly effective for liver and gall-bladder ailments, sluggish digestion, skin conditions, rheumatism, constipation, circulatory and kidney problems.*

ancient times its primary function is still considered to be as a liver, kidney, blood cleansing and digestive tonic. It is regarded as a mild laxative, diuretic, stomachic and tonic, with two especially important functions — to promote the formation of bile and to remove excess water, salt, cholesterol and uric acid from the body.

Dandelion is rich in easily assimilated vitamin complexes and minerals and contains choline, an important B-complex vitamin. The leaves are one of the best natural sources of potassium, and the root contains vitamins A and C and essential fatty acids.

It is frequently used in the treatment of jaundice, cholecystitis (inflammation of the gallbladder), cholelithiasis (stones in the bile duct or gallbladder), hepatitis and in the early stages of cirrhosis of the liver, as well as for chronic rheumatism, gout and stiff joints.

Dandelion is often prescribed for indigestion, constipation, fever or insomnia.

**AVAILABLE FORMS:** Dandelion can be used as a decoction, an infusion and as an extract. It is an ingredient of many herbal mixtures, and may also be taken as tablets, capsules or as a coffee substitute.

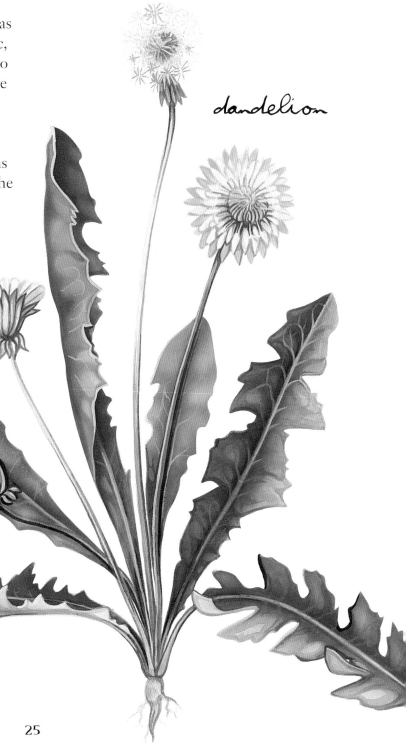

dandelion

# DEVIL'S CLAW

Wood spider, grapple root
*Harpagophytum procumbens*
**FAMILY:** Pedaliaceae

*This powerful plant has stood the test of time in Africa, providing many with the suppleness of body that we in the West strive to keep up in modern times. Devil's claw can get rid of your arthritis, and not a witch doctor in sight.*

**DESCRIPTION:** Devil's claw is a plant native to southwest Africa, growing in the savanna lands of the Kalahari Desert. The fruit is a pod-like capsule, protected by numerous curved spines, which, after splitting out the fruit, take on a claw-like appearance. The plant has fragile, creeping stems; to survive the frequent droughts, it sends down wide, brown, water-storing roots as deep as 3 feet (1 m) into the soil. When the rains come, devil's claw produces spectacular, trumpet-shaped flowers.

**HISTORY:** The African Bushmen have used the plant for thousands of years for digestive problems, rheumatism or sore muscles and limb pains, as well as malaria, fevers, headaches, and general pain or weakness. Not much was known about its use in other parts of the world, until it received acclaim for its pain-reducing and anti-inflammatory effects which resulted in the dramatic recovery of many German soldiers treated by local witch doctors during the Hottentot rebellion in 1904.

When introduced into Europe, it became suddenly famous for its ability to soothe arthritic and rheumatic conditions, migraines, hypertension, fevers and general debility. According to Chinese medicine, devil's claw is both yin and yang, rare in herbal medicine, but extremely beneficial for the circulation and heart.

**MODERN USES:** Devil's claw is the modern-day, natural, analgesic arthritis genie — traditional modern medicine has only been able to come up with aspirin and non-steroidal anti-inflammatory drugs (NSAIDS) as treatment, which can have distinct disadvantages for the rest of your body. Recent studies show that six out of ten arthritic patients will receive significant relief, without side effects, from a course of devil's claw. It acts as a powerful anti-inflammatory agent, reduces pain, swelling and stiffness of inflamed joints and muscles, and has the added bonus of being a liver cleanser and detoxicant of the whole body system. Devil's claw has more than 40 active constituents, all aimed at helping those stiff, sore muscles, joints and bones, and is particularly indicated for fibromyalgia syndrome. It is also prescribed for dyspepsia, loss of appetite, nausea, digestive disorders, constipation and diarrhea, and many liver and gallbladder problems.

**AVAILABLE FORMS** Devil's claw may be combined with other herbs, such as willow bark, or obtained from your health food store as a tablet, tincture or extract. If you have a serious condition, talk to your naturopathic practitioner about which would be the best form for you.

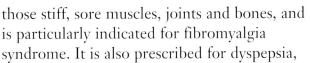

*devil's claw*

*If the pain of arthritis has you firmly in its grip, the anti-inflammatory devil's claw will help ease the pain and swelling.*

# ECHINACEA

Cone flower, Rudbeckia, black sampson
*Echinacea angustifolia*
**FAMILY:** Compositae

*Echinacea is a magnificent herbal antibiotic and blood purifier has become increasingly popular among herbalists and medical practitioners worldwide. It is used mainly to enhance the immune system response.*

**DESCRIPTION:** The cylindrical root system is furrowed, the stem is bristly and stout, the hairy leaves taper at both ends. Echinacea's distinctive flowers feature 12 to 20 large, spreading, rich purple rays with a raised, central, conical disk. Flowering time is from June to October in the northern hemisphere. Medicinally, the rootstock is the most potent part of the plant; it has a faint aromatic smell and a sweetish taste.

**HISTORY:** This native American herbaceous perennial grows from the prairie states northward to the Canadian border. It is now cultivated worldwide for its horticultural beauty and medicinal properties. Native Americans used it as a mouthwash, for poultices and as a health-giving tea. The plant is named after the Greek word for "hedgehog," *Echinos*, referring to the shape of the sharp-pointed leaves. In combination with myrrh, it was said to be useful for typhoid fever. It was commonly used for "conditions of the blood," such as acne, boils, eczema, skin conditions and circulatory problems. In the Middle Ages it was used as an aphrodisiac. Echinacea does not have a widely recorded history, although it was undoubtedly used medicinally; however it has captured public attention in recent times for its success in treating the many modern immune-system disorders.

*There is empirical evidence that echinacea is a great boost for everyone's immune system. Use it to fight infections large or lingering. An efficient and vigilant antiviral, antibacterial blood purifier.*

**MODERN USES:** This revolutionary herb has generated serious interest and research in recent years, since it has been scientifically proven to be a stimulator of the body's immune system, hence building resistance to infections, colds and flu. It is worthwhile taking echinacea with rosehips as a preventive medicine in the fall (autumn) to boost the body's resistance against the ever-increasing common winter illnesses. The extract possesses an interferon-like action, which destroys invading viruses and bacteria and increases the number of white blood cells. It is also used for post-viral syndrome, glandular fever, stress, and chronic fatigue syndrome. Echinacea is a major blood-purifying herb, particularly for boils, eczema, acne, septicemia, liver conditions and rheumatism. It has a tonic effect on the lymphatic system and glands, as it promotes the production of antibodies. Any immune system disorder will be assisted by echinacea's strengthening properties.

**AVAILABLE FORMS:** Take as a decoction, tincture, extract, tablet, infusion or capsule, or grow your own as garden or container plants. It may be topically applied as an ointment, cream or poultice.

*echinacea*

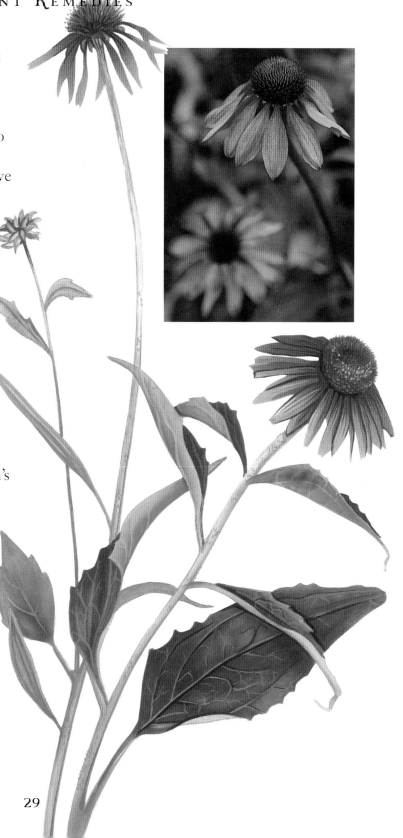

# ELDER FLOWER

Elder, black elder, European elder
*Sambucus nigra*
FAMILY: Caprifoliaceae

*The elder tree has a history as long as it is tall. It has been revered since early times as a provider of health for all who partook of its treasured wine and its curative powers.*

DESCRIPTION: The elder tree is a small shrub or tree which grows to 33 feet (10 m). The leaves are of a deep green. The flowers are flat-topped masses of creamy white, fragrant blossoms, followed by large, drooping bunches of purplish black juicy berries. The elder tree grows in Britain and from Scandinavia to the coast of Africa, generally in moist, shady places, and is now cultivated for its many beneficial properties.

HISTORY: The elder has always been associated with protective magic. Elder wood was thought variously to be the wood of the Cross and of the tree from which Judas hanged himself; it was commonly believed that the branches had the power to ward off witches.

All parts of the tree are useful; in fact, it was long known as "the medicine chest of the country people." An infusion of the bitter leaves was often applied as an insect repellent. The external bark was administered as a purgative in Hippocrates' time, and a soothing skin ointment was made from the green inner bark; the flowers were widely used for freckles, skin conditions and sunburn, and to aid longevity. The berries were a staple ingredient for the Romans as a black hair dye, or used internally for colic and diarrhea. Elderberry wine has been made for centuries for its many healing qualities.

MODERN USES: Elder flowers are used in ointments and creams to relieve chapped skin and as a water extract for eye lotions, being mildly astringent and stimulating.

Quantities of berries should not be eaten as they have a strong purgative effect, but can be cooked in jams and jellies. The primary actions of elder flowers are anticatarrhal, astringent and diaphoretic. Its secondary actions are as an anti-inflammatory and antirheumatic. It is helpful for all mucous membrane problems associated with the sinuses, nose and throat.

Elder is used for rheumatic disorders, fibromyalgia syndrome, the common cold, influenza, chronic nasal catarrh with deafness, sinusitis, inflammations, burns, erysipelas (a skin condition characterized by inflammation, redness and fever) and eye inflammations. A tincture of the young bark relieves asthmatic symptoms and coughs in children. The leaves and flowers are used in an ointment for bruises, hemorrhoids, sprains and chilblains; and tea made from the flowers will promote perspiration in those suffering from colds and fevers.

**AVAILABLE FORMS:** Use the leaves as a fresh leaf ointment or infusion, the flowers as tea, jams, and the berries as wine, jams, or jellies. The roots will make a tea or decoction for digestive disorders.

*All parts of the tree — flowers, bark, leaves, roots and berries — have always enjoyed a prestigious reputation in both ancient and modern medicines.*

*From before the days of Hippocrates, the magical elder has been used for its many medicinal properties.*

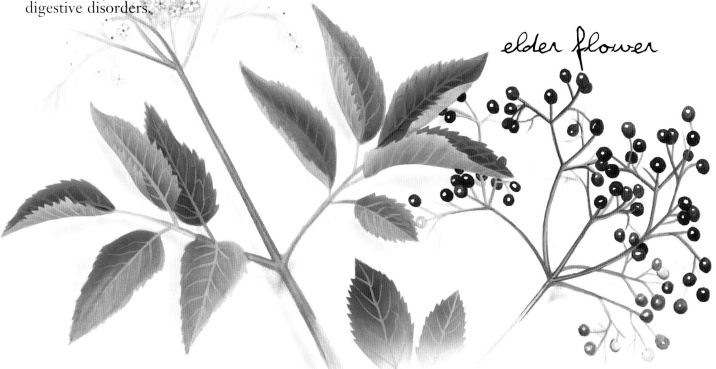

elder flower

# FEVERFEW

Featherfew, pyrethrum parthenium, flirtwort, bachelor's buttons
*Tanacetum parthenium*
**FAMILY:** Compositae

*Feverfew was greatly appreciated as a general tonic in ages past. Its common name is taken from the Latin* **febrifugia**, *meaning a substance that gives flight to fevers.*

**DESCRIPTION:** A perennial, sometimes biennial herbaceous plant, growing to 3 feet (90 cm). Feverfew's hairy, round branching stem bears delicate, yellow green, strongly scented alternate, downy leaves. It has many wide daisy-like flowers, consisting of yellow disk florets with 10–20 white toothed rays in tight clusters. They appear from mid-summer to mid-fall (mid-autumn). Its appearance is similar to chamomile; however, the whole plant has quite a bitter smell, particularly disliked by bees.

*Feverfew has been under the microscope as a migraine-sufferer's salvation. If feverfew is taken as a preventive in sensible doses, the severity and frequency of migraines can be reduced — a welcome relief for anyone who has struggled through the terrible pain.*

**HISTORY:** Feverfew is extensively cultivated in many parts of Canada and America. In Britain, as a cottage-garden plant, it was introduced long ago as a domestic medicine and now grows wild in hedgerows and stone walls all over northern Europe. Traditionally, the herb was planted around dwellings to purify the atmosphere and ward off diseases. John Gerard, in his sixteenth-century *Herball*, spoke highly of its ability to defy ague if placed on the wrists, and as being of great benefit to those sensitive to pain. For many centuries, feverfew has been employed to treat severe headaches and migraines. A decoction was administered for easing coughs, wheezing, depression and breathing difficulties. Earaches were relieved by a cold infusion, while a tincture was traditionally applied to ease the pain and swelling from insect or vermin bites.

**MODERN USES:** Feverfew is an effective preventive remedy against migraine headaches.

Its primary actions are as an antispasmodic, bitter tonic, purgative, menstrual flow stimulator and expectorant. Its secondary actions are as an appetite stimulant, carminative and wound healer, and it can be used effectively for general low spirits, depression or the morning-after effects of alcohol. Its success in migraine therapy is due to its ability to relax smooth-muscle spasms. It contains a compound that assists in controlling the expansion and contraction of blood vessels in the brain, which often cause the associated traumatic symptoms of throbbing head pain and sensitivity to light. Biochemical analysis of the plant has revealed that many migraine sufferers find a significant reduction in pain and/or the frequency of attacks after a short course of treatment. Feverfew has been shown to affect the clotting components of the blood, so anyone with a blood-clotting disorder should probably avoid it without medical supervision.

**AVAILABLE FORMS:** Feverfew can be purchased as tea, infusion, tablets, capsules, tincture or extract. It may be added to the bath for general aches and pains. Feverfew is best avoided in pregnancy.

*feverfew*

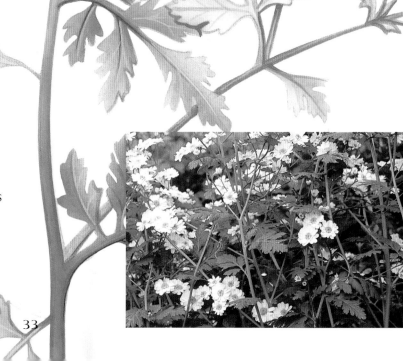

# GARLIC

Poor man's treacle, the stinking rose, Russian penicillin
*Allium sativum*
**FAMILY:** Liliaceae

*"A herb of Mars ... performs almost miracles in phlegmatic habits of the body" – Culpepper*
*And a little miracle herb it has proved itself to be.*

**DESCRIPTION:** Garlic is a perennial herb, belonging to the same group of plant as the onion. The bulb is compound, with many individual cloves enclosed together in a whitish skin. The stem is simple, smooth and round, surrounded at the base by long, flat, grass-like leaf sheaths, leading to a globular head of small, usually sterile white flowers containing 20–30 small bulbils.

**HISTORY:** A plant of great antiquity, garlic was recorded first by the Sumerians about 5,000 years ago. The name was derived from *gar* (a spear) and *lac* (a plant), referring to the shape of its leaves. It was used by the Vikings, Greeks, Egyptians and Babylonians, and was mentioned in several Old English records of plants from the tenth to fifteenth centuries.

The gypsies worshipped it for its medicinal powers, and it has been long employed to ward off evil. There is a Mohammedan legend that "When Satan stepped out from the Garden of Eden after the fall of Man, garlick sprang up from the spot where he placed his left foot, and onion from that where his right foot touched." The builders of the pyramids, and

Greek and Roman soldiers were issued a daily ration of garlic as it was regarded as a valuable strengthening medicine and a potent protection against disease.

**MODERN USES:** Extensive testing on garlic has revealed its ability to lower cholesterol and protect against hypertension and arteriosclerosis, helping to reduce the risk of cardiovascular disease. It is a valuable natural antibiotic for many types of bacterial infection and is administered to cleanse wounds, to combat all types of infection, and to assist in the treatment of viral infections. It is frequently used in combination with echinacea and vitamin C. Garlic is a potent antiseptic blood purifier and is beneficial as a decongestant and expectorant, preventing and relieving chronic bronchitis, sinusitis, hay fever, colds and flu, and stomach and intestinal catarrh. It also regulates liver function and assists many skin conditions, such as cold sores, herpes, boils, impetigo and some allergies. Rich in sulfur, garlic is also good for the garden, encouraging growth in other plants — especially roses. Spread powdered garlic or spray around seedlings to protect them against birds, small creatures and insects.

**AVAILABLE FORMS:** Garlic may be purchased from the supermarket, or you may grow it yourself. Crush the cloves and apply externally as an ointment, lotion or poultice. Include fresh cloves or juice in your salad dressings and cooking. Garlic can also be purchased in the form of a tincture, an extract, gelatin oil capsule or tablet.

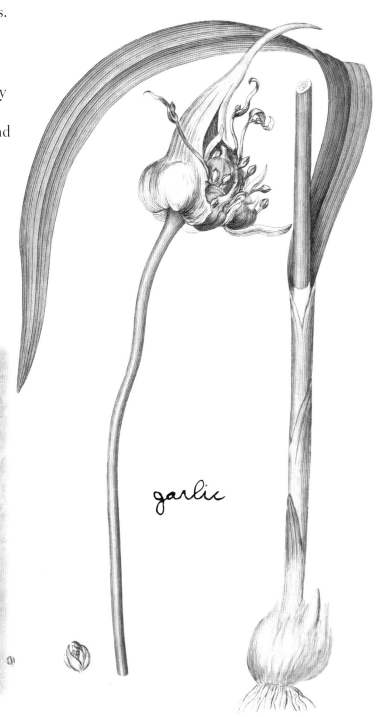

garlic

*Garlic is a culinary and medicinal acrobat. Its historical range of application in the kitchen, the medicine cabinet and the garden has made an enticing attraction for humankind on the one hand, and a rigorous repeller of disease on the other.*

# GENTIAN

Bitterwort, yellow gentian
*Gentiana lutea*
FAMILY: Gentianaceae

*Gentian "comforts the heart and preserves it against faintings and swoonings: the powder of the dry roots helps the biting of mad dogs and venomous beasts ..." – Culpepper*

DESCRIPTION: A hardy and ornamental perennial growing to 3 feet (90 cm) on a thick tap root that can be 2 feet (60 cm) long, gentian has shiny, oval leaves 1 foot (30 cm) in length and 6 inches (15 cm) wide. It has attractive, bright yellow flowers 1¹/2 inches (3 cm) long in 3–10 flowered clusters, which appear in the late summer to early fall (autumn), but generally not until the plants are about ten years old.

*Gentian is a lifesaver for people with slow digestive systems and those who eat a lot of fast food. When eating on the run, gentian can help revive you after rich or heavy meals.*

HISTORY: Gentian is a native of the alpine and sub-alpine pastures of southern Europe, and is now frequently found in most temperate regions of the world. The name is derived from Gentius, an ancient king of Illyria who reigned in180 B.C. and who, according to Pliny and Dioscorides, discovered the medicinal powers of the plant. During the Middle Ages, gentian was frequently employed as a somewhat bitter antidote to many poisons. According to Culpepper, "'tis very wholesome, but not very toothsome." Before being superseded by hops, gentian was used to make beer and tonic, and it has long been used to make bitter aperitifs in France. It has been employed for over 2,000 years as a fortifying tonic and a treatment for fever, most digestive troubles and, externally, as an antiseptic herb to apply on wounds.

MODERN USES: Like all bitter plants, gentian acts as a tonic for the whole digestive system. Primarily, it is a strong, bitter-tasting tonic that increases salivary flow, stomach secretions and bile flow. The latter two functions help to increase appetite and improve digestion. It is administered for indigestion, anorexia, diarrhea and vomiting. Gentian's secondary actions are as an antispasmodic, antiseptic, menstrual-flow stimulant and febrifuge; it can be beneficial for tiredness or general apathy, loss of appetite and any immune system breakdown, due to its ability to raise the white blood cell count. It helps liver disorders, nausea, dyspepsia, stomach ulcers, jaundice nd biliousness and is also used for anti-inflammatory and arthritic conditions, including fibromyalgia syndrome and sciatica. The fresh leaves can be placed directly on wounds as a soothing agent, and can be added to a foot bath or sitz bath to provide a healing balm for varicose veins and hemorrhoids.

**AVAILABLE FORMS:** Gentian is available as a tincture, fluid extract, tea, tablet, capsule or fresh herb. It is often included in digestive compounds. In general, it should be taken half an hour before eating.

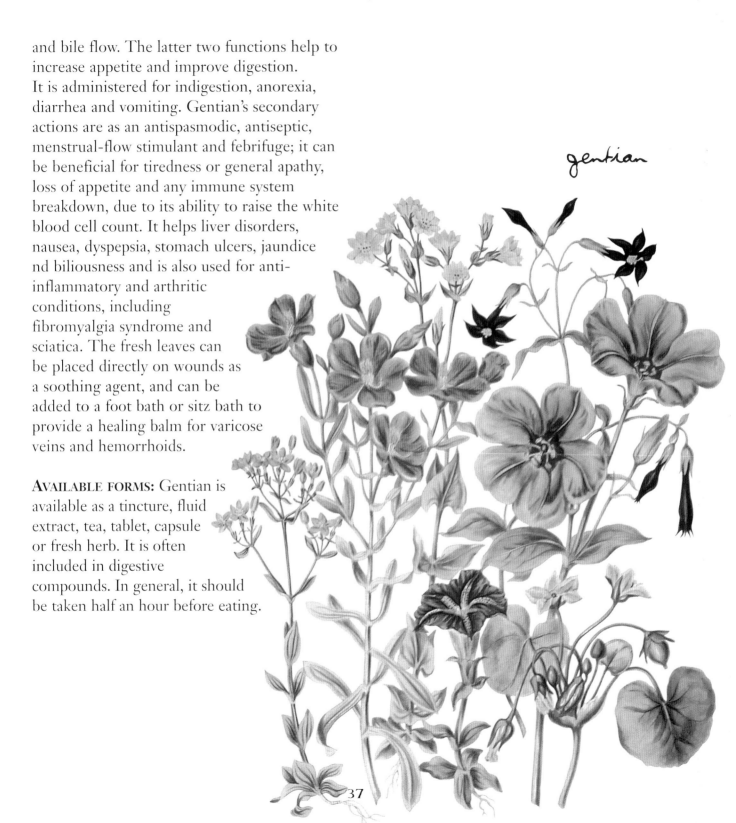

gentian

# GINGER

Jamaica ginger, black ginger
*Zingiber officinale*
FAMILY: Zingiberaceae

*Ginger was one of the most popular spices in medieval cookery — its warming, rich and pungent flavor is still much in favor today.*

**DESCRIPTION:** The aromatic, knotted ginger rhizome, which creeps and expands underground, is thick, fibrous and, externally, a buff to light brown color. The root produces a simple, leafy stalk, 2–3 feet (60–90 cm) high, with narrow oblong leaves, 6–12 inches (15–30 cm) long, which lie dormant annually. The flowering stalk shoots straight up from the root, ending in an oblong spike, from which a sterile yellow or white and purple flower grows.

*Ginger has a history of culinary and medicinal application. Imported from Asia by the ancient Greeks, it has kept its place as an important adjunct to modern medicine. It is a warming stimulant and an active system cleanser.*

**HISTORY:** Ginger is a perennial plant indigenous to Southeast Asia, cultivated in many tropical areas of the world, especially Jamaica, and brought to America by the Spaniards. It was imported from Asia by the ancient Greeks and has been part of daily life in Asia for centuries, where it is still an important ingredient in Chinese medicine. Ginger tea was used in Old England as an infusion for "stoppage of the menses," digestive and liver conditions, and, externally, for promoting blood supply to areas of poor circulation and rheumatism. The tea was used as a stimulant at the onset of a cold, frequently in combination with peppermint and cayenne. Chinese medicine has held ginger in high regard and it was used through the ages as a therapy for all stomach conditions.

**MODERN USES:** Ginger's medicinal applications are still primarily as a carminative, stimulant and antispasmodic. It is of particular benefit to the stomach, intestines and circulation. Its warming, relaxing properties make it helpful in flatulent colic, dyspepsia, nausea, diarrhea — where there is no

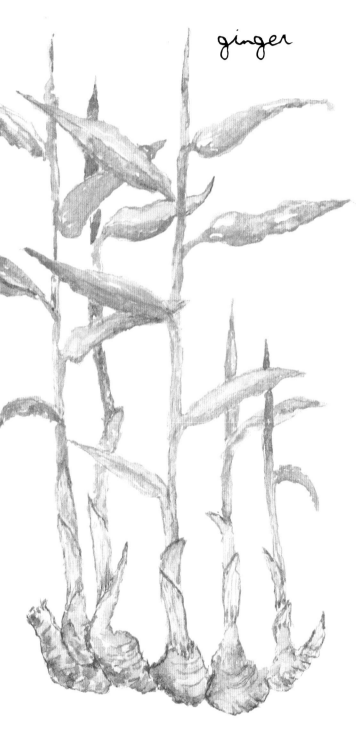

ginger

inflammation — and underactive digestion. It is often an ingredient in herbal compounds for suppressed or painful menstruation. Ginger stimulates the production of saliva, which in turn stimulates gastric-acid secretion. It is also particularly beneficial for colds, chills and influenza, as it enhances cleansing of the system by promoting perspiration. It is also known to assist the action of other herbs. Externally, it may be applied as a compress or in ointment form for the treatment of stiff joints, rheumatism, inflammation and pain. Chewing a piece of the root helps ease the discomfort of a sore throat.

**AVAILABLE FORMS:** Ginger root may be purchased from your greengrocer or supermarket. Make a hot infusion from ½ oz. (15 g.) of bruised or powdered root added to 1 pint (600 ml) of boiling water, with 1 oz. (30 g.) being taken two or three times daily. Tinctures, tablets, capsules, and essential oil of ginger are available from health food stores. In tincture form, ginger should be taken as 20 drops in a little water, before meals.

# GINKGO

Maidenhair tree
*Ginkgo biloba*
FAMILY: Ginkgoacea

*The maidenhair tree has been recognized as the modern savior of the brain —*
*particularly when it comes to preventing cerebral degeneration associated*
*with aging and memory loss.*

DESCRIPTION: Ginkgoes grow to 100 feet (30 m). Deciduous, with unusual, feathery, fan-shaped leaves that yellow in the fall (autumn), the trees are male or female — with the males producing spikes of yellow flowers; females, acorn-like flowers. Ginkgoes grow slowly, but when in their maturity, majesty prevails. They prefer moist soil and moderate to cool climates. As a garden tree, buy a grafted female, as the fruit of the male dispels a pervading, unpleasant odor.

HISTORY: Ginkgoes have survived for 200 million years and are possibly the world's oldest living tree. They have endured major climate changes, including several ice ages, and have developed a resistance to most pollution, pests, fungi and native wildlife.

They are native to China and Japan, and were imported to Europe in the eighteenth century, where they have assumed a prominent position in horticultural landscapes. The Chinese used ginkgo internally for lung conditions and externally on the kidney acupuncture meridians, for incontinence, excessive urination and cystitis. The ginkgo is the only tree of its kind, with just one species grown throughout the world in mild climates. The fruit of the male ginkgo has long been considered a delicacy in Asia.

MODERN USES: The leaves are harvested in the fall (autumn) to extract their main active pharmacological substance, whose target organ is the brain. Ginkgo promotes better blood circulation throughout the body but especially to the brain, and simultaneously increases absorption of carbohydrates, essential for proper brain function. Its free-radical-scavenging effect, combined with its action on blood vessels and ability to increase metabolic processes during decreased blood supply, suggest it may be effective in arterial insufficiency, hardening of the arteries, tiredness, anxiety, apathy and some cancerous conditions. Ginkgo also offers protection against, and helps with recovery from, strokes. Patients with cerebral vascular insufficiency who suffer from short-term memory loss, vertigo, headache, ringing in the ears, and depression have benefited from taking ginkgo, and it is being investigated extensively in the treatment of Alzheimer's disease and dementia. Because of its proven track record with aging-related cerebral dysfunction, ginkgo has received a lot of positive publicity.

**AVAILABLE FORMS:** You can purchase ginkgo as a fresh-leaf tea, as tablets, capsules, extracts, tinctures, or you can grow your own "tree of remembrance."

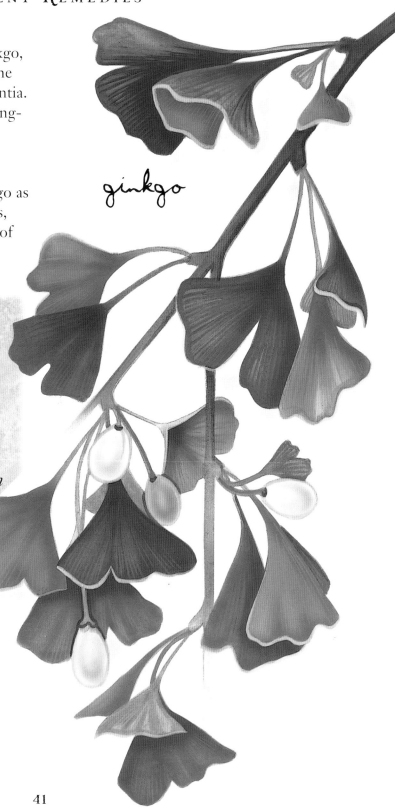

ginkgo

*Benefit from the antiaging*

*properties of the tree which itself has*

*survived for 200 million years.*

*Ginkgo may help your mental function*

*and extend your life.*

# GINSENG

American ginseng, five-fingers, man's health
*Panax ginseng*
FAMILY: Araliaceae

*Ginseng is a universal panacea, aphrodisiac and elixir. It appears to adapt to the needs of the body, strengthening all its parts and prolonging life. Ginseng seems to be the ultimate tonic medicine.*

DESCRIPTION: The seeds generally take nearly two years to germinate. The fleshy root produces a few leaves with five leaflets, and small greenish yellow flowers in mid-summer followed by bright red berries. It is ready for harvesting after six years.

Ginseng measures up to 2 feet (60 cm) long and is often shaped roughly like a human form.

*The ultimate tonic-for-all-occasions, ginseng is a "pick me up" during extended periods of stress and anxiety. It can increase mental, physical and sexual energy, and if used wisely, prevents feelings of lethargy.*

HISTORY: Ginseng grows in woodlands in eastern North America, and was imported to Europe in the early 1700s. The name "ginseng" comes from the Chinese word meaning "man-shape," referring to the root's human-like form, although a widespread usage has it meaning "the wonder of the world." Panax, the generic name, comes from the Greek *panakos*, a panacea, for the widespread belief in its wondrous virtues for almost all diseases. A similar species, Chinese ginseng, has been used medicinally in China and Tibet since about 3,000 B.C., and is particularly indicated for dyspepsia, vomiting, nervous disorders, apathy, depression and stress. Native Americans took a liquified form of ginseng to relieve nausea and vomiting, and it has been administered in many cultures as an ingredient in love potions and as a sexual stimulant.

MODERN USES: The primary uses of ginseng are as a herb which can adapt to the body's needs, as an adrenal stimulant, a metabolic stimulant, a reproductive and sexual stimulator, and in general, a whole-body tonic and

restorative. The general indicators for its use are any digestive disorders aggravated by mental or nervous stress, including diarrhea, nausea, ulcers, indigestion, appetite loss, weight loss or gain, immune system disorders and fatigue.
There are various species of ginseng, and most are used as general tonics, especially recommended for apathy and debility, for mental and nervous exhaustion, stress, depression — especially in cases of sexual inadequacy — insomnia, and memory loss. It is also utilized as a general nerve tonic and as an antioxidant, assisting in heart and circulatory problems, including hypertension, varicose veins, liver or kidney weakness, and chronic respiratory problems.

**AVAILABLE FORMS:** Tablets, capsules, fluid essences, extracts, powder and teas.

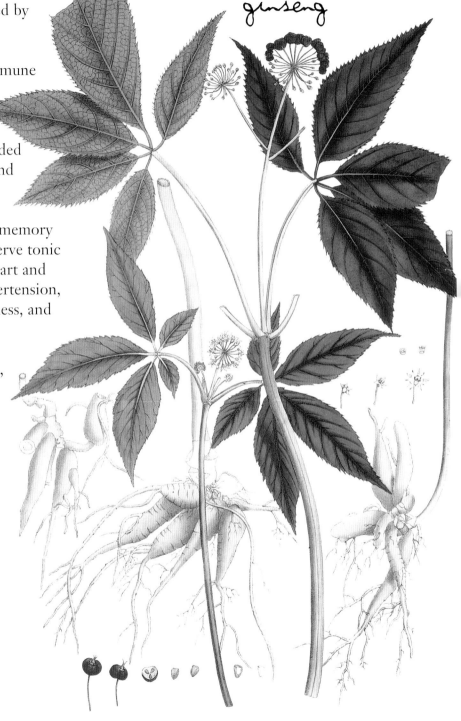

ginseng

# HORSE CHESTNUT

Buckeye, Spanish chestnut
*Aesculus hippocastanum*
FAMILY: Hippocastanaceae

*Another of Nature's medicine chests, this beautiful tree provides
medicines from all its parts, for most of ours.*

DESCRIPTION: The deciduous horse chestnut tree grows from 50–80 feet (15–24 m) high. The erect trunk grows very rapidly, with widely spreading branches. Unusual markings, in the shape of miniature horseshoes, can be found all over the small branches. Its bark is grayish green in color and smooth, and its large leaves are divided into five to seven finely toothed leaflets. The flowers are white, reddish or yellow, and the prickly green globular fruit capsule contains from one to six shiny brown seeds.

*Horse chestnut can help with a variety of modern-day conditions, from varicose veins, hemorrhoids, strains and sprains, to many internal conditions, including bronchitis, colds, the flu and diarrhea.*

HISTORY: The horse chestnut tree is a native of Europe and Asia, introduced into England in about the middle of the sixteenth century, and now commonly cultivated in America and Canada. It is not related to the sweet chestnut — however its name "horse" may be a corruption of the Welsh *gwres*, meaning hot, fierce or pungent — in contrast to the qualities of the mild, sweet one. Traditionally, European folk medicine extolled the benefits of carrying the fruit in one's pocket to prevent or cure arthritis. It was employed all over the world for treating varicose veins and hemorrhoids, for its general anti-inflammatory properties, and as a sunscreen. The bark was utilized in treating fevers, asthma and bronchitis, and the fruit in the treatment of rheumatism and neuralgia.

MODERN USES: Today, horse chestnut is most valued for its use in treating varicose veins, hemorrhoids, enlargement of the prostate, menstrual cramps, rheumatism, diarrhea, sciatica, fevers and the symptoms of the common cold. It is also an effective expectorant for bronchitis, catarrh and asthma. Because it

44

has astringent and diuretic qualities, it is also helpful for many skin conditions, kidney disorders and fluid retention. Modern research has revealed that horse chestnut is effective in relieving the painful symptoms of cystitis. It is used topically for any soft tissue injuries, sunburn, and painful conditions of the joints, ligaments or tendons, such as sciatica, fibromyalgia, sprains or strains (particularly when there is inflammation). It has been shown to be helpful in the treatment of leg ulcers, bruises and leg cramps — however, it should not be used on broken skin or in large doses.

**AVAILABLE FORMS:** Fluid extracts, decoctions, infusions, tablets, compounds are all available from your health food store. Ask your naturopath which is the most suitable form for you — the fresh fruit and seeds can be poisonous, so don't take them internally without medical advice.

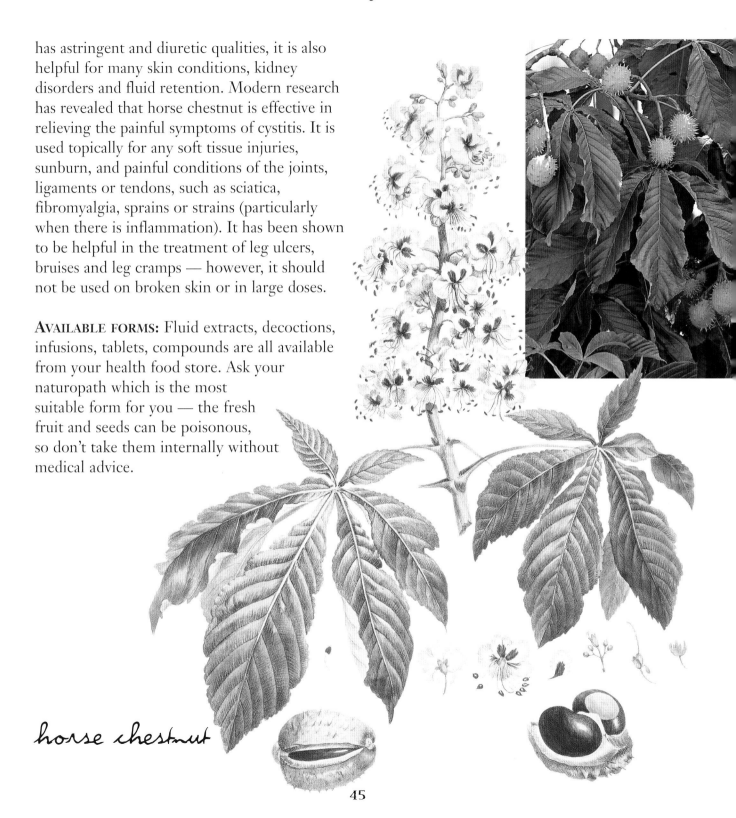

*horse chestnut*

45

# LICORICE

Licorice root, sweet licorice, sweetwood
*Glycyrrhiza glabra*
FAMILY: Leguminosae

*One of the world's most widely known herbs, licorice has a history that dates back centuries in both Eastern and Western cultures. It has been used since the third century B.C. for almost everything that ails the human form.*

**DESCRIPTION:** Licorice is a perennial herb with a stem 2–5 feet (0.6–1.6 m) tall, rising from a thick woody root. The narrow, long, dark green leaves have four to seven pairs of feathery, drooping leaflets. The flower is yellowish white or purple, followed by small pods resembling a partly grown pea pod. The fruit is a brown legume, 1 inch (2.5 cm) long. The medicinal cylindrical tap root often grows 6–8 inches (14–20 cm) long and 2–8 inches (5–20 cm) wide.

**HISTORY:** In the third century B.C., the Greek philosopher Theophrastus observed that chewing a piece of licorice would prevent thirst. Dioscorides named the plant Glycyrrhiza from the Greek *glukos* meaning "sweet," and *riza*, "a root," in recognition of its sweet taste. Licorice was widely used in Europe during the Middle Ages and was recorded as a general digestive tonic in Germany in the eleventh century. In 1264, licorice was regarded as being of great value to the court of Henry IV. Serious cultivation of the herb began in the early sixteenth century.

*Licorice — the sweetest herb around — is a soother, tonic and restorative blood cleanser all in one.*

In traditional Chinese medicine, licorice assists the twelve primary meridians, especially the spleen and lung. It replenishes chi (the life force), clears heat, strengthens the lungs, controls coughs, harmonizes the stomach and spleen, detoxifies drugs, soothes spasms and acts as an antidote to body toxins.

**MODERN USES:** Licorice is an excellent expectorant for treating coughs, colds, bronchial congestion, hoarseness, mild fevers and mucous congestion. It is a soothing and restorative remedy for sore throats or laryngitis, as well as being a mild laxative that can be given to children and anyone with constipation, appetite loss or who is feeling tired or depressed. The Chinese use licorice to counteract infections, and in many cultures it is utilized to protect the liver and kidneys. Its anti-inflammatory action is employed to treat stomach and intestinal ulcers. As a cautionary note, frequent or large doses of licorice may cause sodium retention and potassium loss, leading to high blood pressure, fluid retention, headache, diarrhea and shortness of breath. Licorice contains substances similar to estrogen-like compounds and the adrenocortical hormones, and for this reason, it is useful for adrenal insufficiency and other hormonal or immune system problems. Its estrogenic properties make it helpful during menopause and its action on the adrenal glands improves the ability to resist stress.

**AVAILABLE FORMS:** Licorice can be purchased at health food stores in many forms — powdered root, decoction, tincture, extract, tea, capsule, tablet and candy.

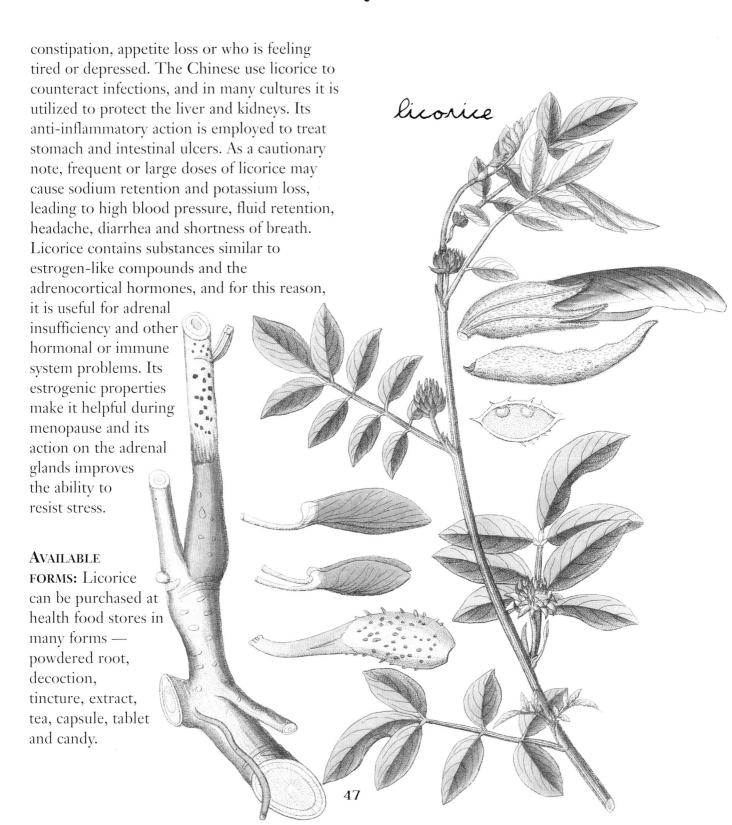

licorice

# MARSHMALLOW

Sweet weed, Schloss tea, Althea
*Althaea officinalis*
**FAMILY:** Malvaceae

*All mallows, including the garden hollyhock, contain quantities of mucilage, and the marshmallow is an especially soothing healing herb.*

**DESCRIPTION:** Marshmallow is a sprawling plant, growing to about 3 feet (1 m) high. The stem and large, irregularly toothed lobed leaves are covered with a soft, velvet down. The pale pink flowers bloom in late summer, followed by fruits (historically called "cheeses" because of their round, flattened shape), with long, cream-colored perennial roots, thick, tapering and very tough and fibrous both inside and out.

**HISTORY:** Marshmallow generally grows near the sea, by river estuaries and in salt marshes in Britain, Europe, and America, and is said to have been first introduced by the Romans. The herb is an eastern European native, which was brought to the American, Australian and New Zealand colonies by the early settlers. Its generic name, Althaea, comes from the Greek, *altho*, "to cure" and its family name, Malvaceae, from the Greek, *malake*, "to soften." It was consumed as a food, especially with sweetmeats, and was also used medicinally in poultices, ointments and infusions. The ancient Greeks spoke of the laxative abilities of the root, and the early Arab physicians extolled its virtues as a poultice to suppress inflammation and for the treatment of cuts and wounds.

**MODERN USES:** Marshmallow is a demulcent, emollient and diuretic herb. Its particular ability is to soothe irritated tissue. Internally, its demulcent properties will soothe inflamed

*The powerful demulcent and emollient properties of marshmallow make it renowned as the great soother for any inflammatory disorders or irritation of the digestive tract.*

gastric mucous membranes. Externally, it can be used as a poultice for irritations, burns, carbuncles, boils and wounds. An infusion of the leaves and flowers makes a soothing, relieving gargle. A decoction of the root makes a good vaginal douche or a soothing eyewash.

The cold extract of the root or the whole plant as a tea alleviates cystitis, coughing, whooping cough, catarrh, colds and bronchitis. Inhale steam containing marshmallow leaves for sinusitis and colds. Marshmallow can help in many digestive problems and can be taken for nausea, indigestion, colitis and ulcers. It is often given to children and infants in syrup form, frequently in combination with licorice. Marshmallow is used to make fine-grade soaps and creams for irritated skin, and a decoction of the roots and leaves is often included in lotions for burns, sores, sunburn, and dry skin. Most benefit is obtained from decoctions, teas and ointments.

**AVAILABLE FORMS:** Decoctions, teas, ointments, lotions, creams, infusions, syrup, tincture and poultices are available at health food stores and from some pharmacies.

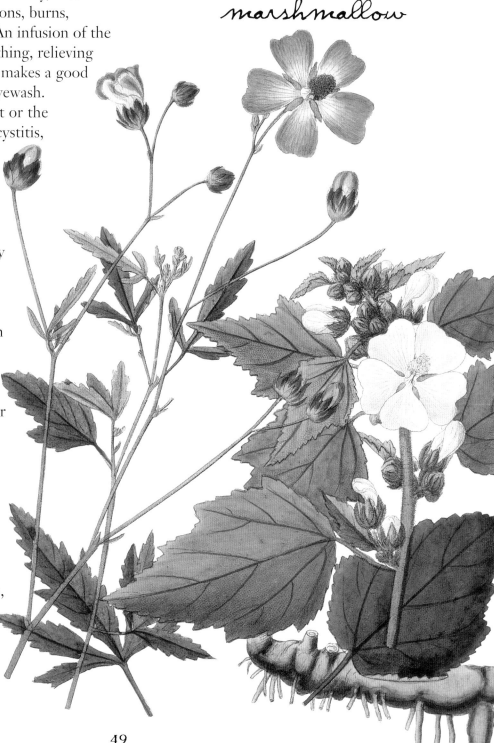

marshmallow

# MEADOWSWEET

Lady of the meadow, midwest, queen of the meadow, bridewort
*Filipendula ulmaria*
**FAMILY:** Rosaceae

*"Makes the heart merry and joyful and delighteth the senses" — John Gerard*
*Meadowsweet is used for stomach problems, fevers,*
*urinary tract infections and rheumatism.*

*Meadowsweet was the first plant in which salicylic acid was found, and from which aspirin was later synthesized, hence its status as a mild, organic alternative for pain, fevers and rheumatism.*

**DESCRIPTION:** Meadowsweet, a perennial herb, thrives in damp fields and woods throughout Europe, America and Canada. Growing 2–4 feet (60–120 cm) tall with fern-like leaves, it has strawberry red to creamy white flowers, which have an almond-like fragrance; there is also a pink flowering variety. The leaves are irregular with a serrated, downy, white underside, resembling those of the elm (*Ulmus*), hence the species name, *ulmaria*.

**HISTORY:** Meadowsweet, watermint and vervain were the three herbs most sacred to the Druids, who used the flowers to flavor wine, beer and mead, hence its original name, "meadwort." The fresh flowers were boiled with water to treat ague and diarrhea, and to bathe sore eyes. They were also used for stomach aches and children's ailments such as colic or mild stomach aches. Meadowsweet was mixed with copper to make a strong black dye. Originally the herb was classified *Spiraea ulmaria* by Linnaeus because of the sweet-smelling fruit spirals and twists around the leaves. Culpepper warned that "the leaves, when they are full grown, being laid on the skin will, in a short time, raise blisters." Meadowsweet was the first plant in which salicylic acid was discovered (in 1839), and from which our modern drug aspirin (named from *Spiraea*) was later synthesized.

**MODERN USES:** Meadowsweet is used to treat peptic ulcers. It normalizes stomach function and is one of the best remedies for hyperacidity and heartburn. It is also used for treating vomiting and diarrhea, especially in children. Due to its salicylate content, it can reduce mild fevers and flu symptoms and assist with rheumatic, gouty joints and many types of muscular pain. It has diuretic and antiseptic properties suitable for the treatment of kidney and bladder infections, fluid retention and cellulitis.

To enhance the complexion, the flowers should be soaked in water for several hours, strained, and the water used as a face (or body) wash. Throw a handful of the fragrant flowers into the bath, along with some chamomile flowers, to help reduce stress levels. Make a cold compress from the flowers for external swelling and inflammation.

**AVAILABLE FORMS:** Health food stores should stock meadowsweet in some or all of the following forms: liquid extract, tincture, powder, infusion, tea, and as a fresh herb.

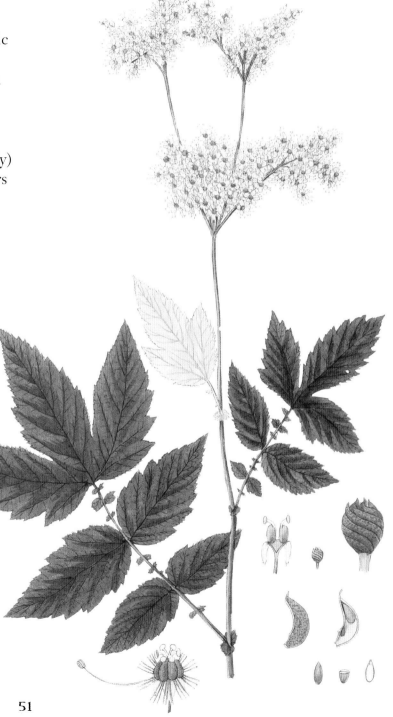

*meadowsweet*

# MILK THISTLE

Marian thistle, wild artichoke, St. Mary's thistle
*Silybum marianum*
**FAMILY:** Compositae

*The lion at the gates of the liver, milk thistle helps to regenerate liver cells and protects it from excessive damage caused by a variety of ingested toxins.*

**DESCRIPTION:** An annual or biennial plant, milk thistle grows from 1–5 feet (30–150 cm) tall with an erect, prominently grooved, rarely branched stem. The leaves are large, oblong, glossy, variegated and very spiny. Its pretty thistle-like violet to purple flowers grow to 2 inches (5 cm) long, and are usually solitary and surrounded at the base by long, spiny appendages, appearing late summer or early fall (autumn).

**HISTORY:** Milk thistle is found in dry, rocky soils in Europe and in some parts of America. In northern Europe, the milk thistle was thought "a great breeder of milk and a diet for wet nurses." The heads were eaten like those of the artichoke, and the young shoots, stalks and roots considered a fine and nutritious addition to many meals.

It was believed in medieval times that the milk-white veins of the leaves originated in the milk of the Virgin which once fell upon a plant of thistle, hence "St. Mary's Thistle."

Culpepper believed it was a cure for ague and apathy, preventing and curing the infection of the plague, and for removal of

*The great balancing act: Milk thistle can help alleviate depression, repair your liver and purify your blood — with very little effort or fuss.*

obstructions of the liver — including jaundice — and the spleen. He recommended the young plant be eaten as a blood cleanser.

**MODERN USES:** The seeds are effective in treating liver, gall bladder and spleen problems, such as jaundice, gallstone colic and the stimulation of bile flow. They also work preventively against car sickness. The leaves are used for common stomach problems, such as lack of appetite and dyspepsia. John Gerard wrote: "My opinion is that this is the best remedy that grows against all melancholy diseases." (*Melan* is Greek for "black" and *cholia* means "bile.") This is another way of saying it has a therapeutic action on the liver. Milk thistle is a number one hepatoprotectant (liver protector). In times of toxic assault on the body, it will help protect the liver cells. It is recommended during chemotherapy and as a safeguard against damage from excessive alcohol intake, as well as for depression. It works well in companionship with dandelion and globe artichoke for cleansing, rebuilding and protecting the liver and gallbladder.

**AVAILABLE FORMS:** Different parts of the plant need to be taken in different ways, depending on what is to be treated. The seeds should be powdered, then taken in an emulsion. The leaves are best used fresh and dried. Young leaves, shoots, peeled stems, flower heads and roots are cooked and eaten. The fresh plant may be grown, and milk thistle is also available as an extract, tincture and tablet.

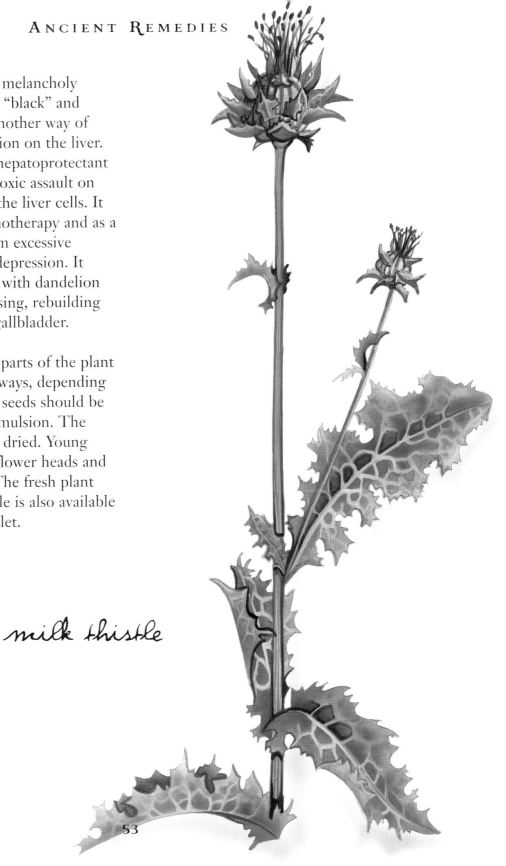

*milk thistle*

# PEPPERMINT

Black peppermint, brandy mint
*Mentha piperita*
**FAMILY:** Labiatae

*This handy and hardy plant produces perhaps
the most widely used and versatile of all the volatile oils.*

**DESCRIPTION:** Peppermint is a hybrid perennial plant found wild in Europe, America and moist temperate regions of the world, though now it is mostly cultivated. Its dark green, serrated leaves are distinctly stalked, 2 inches (5 cm) or more in length with smooth surfaces; the erect, branching stems are 2–4 feet (60–120 cm) high, often purplish in color. The clusters of small reddish violet flowers rarely bear seeds. The entire plant has a strong aromatic menthol odor, caused by the menthol oil it contains.

**HISTORY:** According to Pliny, the Greeks and Romans lived it up in style, with peppermint crowns on their heads and adorning their tables. They also added the herb to their medicines, their foods and wines. Peppermint was mentioned in the Icelandic medical records of the thirteenth century as a digestive tonic, but only came into widespread use in Europe in the seventeenth century, thought to be first used in England. The plant was cultivated extensively in Japan and China (although there is some doubt that it was this exact species), for its chief medicinal constituent, menthol, for which it was commonly utilized in the preparation of oils, ointments and inhalants. It was used in the treatment of many rheumatic, arthritic, muscular pain and respiratory problems.

**MODERN USES:** Peppermint is known to be an anodyne (pain-killer), antispasmodic, carminative, stomachic, cholagogue (bile flow stimulator) and tonic, with an antiseptic action. Peppermint tea or extract can be taken for many stomach and digestive conditions, such as appetite loss, anorexia, colic, indigestion and ulcers; it is also effective in treating insomnia, anxiety and depression as well as sudden pains, cramps, diarrhea or muscular spasms. It can be safely given to children to help digestion and teething problems. The oil can be made into a steam inhalant or added to an oil burner for coughs, colds and flu, or used externally for its

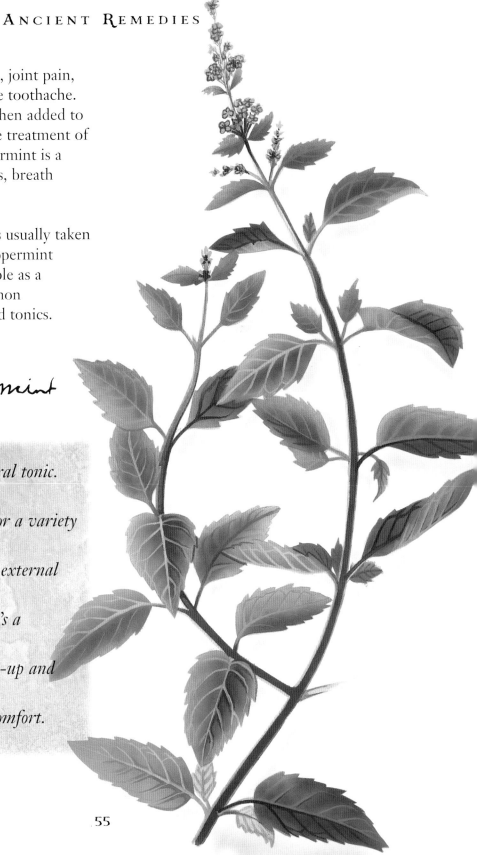

anaesthetic action on rheumatism, joint pain, sciatica and neuralgia or to relieve toothache. The leaves can be very helpful, when added to a bath or made into a salve, in the treatment of any itching skin condition. Peppermint is a frequent ingredient in toothpastes, breath fresheners and cordials.

**AVAILABLE FORMS:** Peppermint is usually taken as tea or infusion, as an oil or peppermint water distillation. It is also available as a tincture or extract, and as a common ingredient in salves, cosmetics and tonics.

*peppermint*

*Peppermint is a good general tonic.*

*Make use of it as treatment for a variety*

*of day-to-day internal and external*

*stresses and strains; it's a*

*great modern-day pick-me-up and*

*will relieve digestive discomfort.*

# PSYLLIUM

Plantago afra, psyllium seed, fleaseed
*Plantago psyllium*
FAMILY: Plantaginaceae

*Psyllium seeds have been around since the time of the ancient Greeks. They are rich in mucilage, and when chewed and swallowed, swell with water to provide comforting relief for many digestive problems.*

DESCRIPTION: There are many varieties of this annual common plant which grows in dry soils all over Europe, northern Africa and Australasia. In general, it is an erect 4–14 inches (10–35 cm) tall plant, bearing long, thin, gray green leaves, with numerous small white to pale yellow flowers. The chewy, mucilaginous seeds are dark brown, convex, shiny and nearly tasteless.

HISTORY: In Scottish history, psyllium was called *slanlus*, a Gaelic word meaning "the plant of healing." It has been used for centuries in many cultures, and Dioscorides recorded that it should be applied as a poultice for every kind of sore, and for relief of toothache. Shakespeare mentions the use of its leaves for broken skin in *Romeo and Juliet*. Its name was derived from the Greek word for flea, *psylla*, because of the seed's flea-like appearance. It has long been held as a powerful healing herb in Europe, India and China, most commonly used for its laxative treatment for chronic constipation or diarrhea — the seed's mucilage swells in water, and the gelatinous mass acts as a bulk purgative. It was frequently applied as a soothing agent for skin conditions, eye irritations and in skin-care preparations.

*Although around since ancient times, scientists are now proving just how much psyllium can help people cope with today's fast-paced lifestyle.*

MODERN USES: In recent times, psyllium seeds have become recognized and incorporated into medicine for their many benefits in our stressful, fast-food-eating lifestyle. Their bulky, mucilaginous benefit comes from their ability to soothe any inflammation or disturbance of the gastrointestinal tract, from mild stomach ache to severe constipation or diarrhea;

psyllium seeds can work as a laxative and to strengthen the digestive tract. Psyllium is frequently prescribed for colitis, irritable bowel syndrome, nausea, ulcers, appetite loss and stress-induced digestive disorders. Recently, it has been shown to help lower blood cholesterol, and is consequently being investigated for possible therapeutic effects on circulatory conditions, liver disorders, allergies and alcohol abuse. It is frequently employed for its benefits in the reproductive and urinary system, especially for its soothing effects in cystitis and, often in combination with herbs such as marshmallow and raspberry leaf, for menstrual cramps. The leaves can be applied externally and some preparations are used for eye lotions, insect bites and wounds.

**AVAILABLE FORMS:** Seeds can be purchased at health food stores and taken as a daily supplement. Preparations that contain psyllium seeds used to soothe skin irritations are also available.

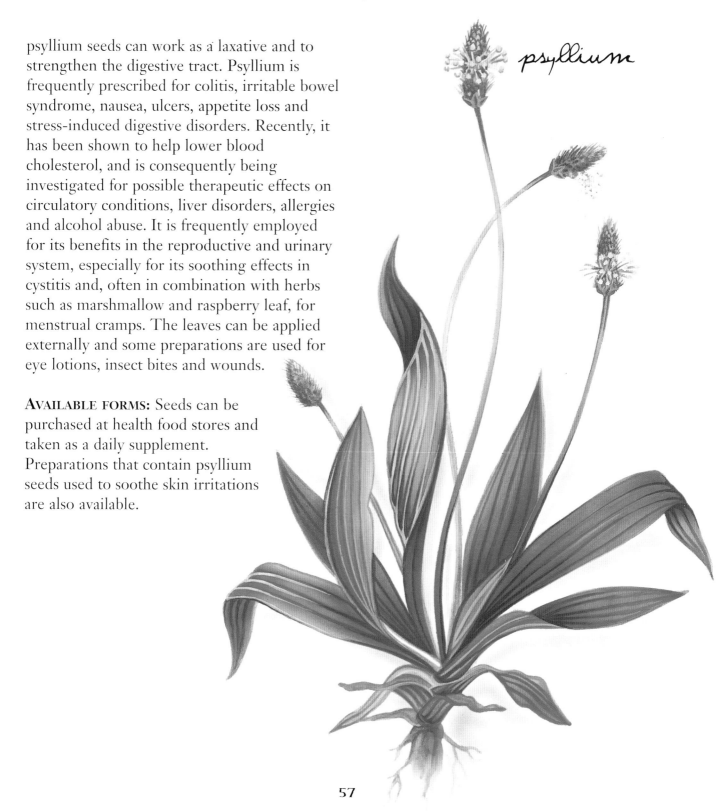

*psyllium*

# RASPBERRY LEAF

Garden raspberry, red raspberry, bramble of Mount Ida
*Rubus idaeus*
**FAMILY:** Rosaceae

*Apart from its value as a sweet, delicious and sensual fruit, the common raspberry also provides us with ingredients for the home medicine chest.*

**DESCRIPTION:** Famous for its delicious fruit, the biennial raspberry plant may be either stooped or erect, and is generally 3–5 feet (90–150 cm) tall, with creeping perennial roots. It has shrubby stems with or without prickles, and its small clusters of 1–6 white, cup-shaped flowers appear early to mid summer, followed by the aromatic, cone-shaped, fleshy red fruit.

**HISTORY:** The raspberry's name, used by the ancient Greeks and Romans, reflects its ancient origins — *rubus* from the Latin for red and *idaea* from Mount Ida in Asia Minor, where it grew profusely from early recorded history. In Europe, cultivation began on a serious scale in the Middle Ages, where it became commonly used as a tea, gargle or infusion for colds, coughs, sore throats, teeth or gums, stomach complaints and diarrhea, and as a tonic for pregnancy, childbirth, and postpartum recovery. Externally, it was traditionally applied to burns and scalds to promote healing, for cleansing wounds, and as a diluted wash for ulcers and skin irritations.

Throughout many cultures and centuries, it was employed as a home remedy in the form of teas, jams, wines, foods and vinegars.

**MODERN USES:** Today, raspberry leaf is best known for its astringent, tonic, stimulant, as well as relaxant properties. It is utilized for all sorts of women's conditions — regular use of the tea should help provide a trouble-free pregnancy, due to, among other factors, the herb's high folic acid, iron, vitamins A and C content.

Raspberry strengthens the pelvic muscles and ligaments, helps ward off morning

*The gentle raspberry leaf has long been considered a particularly useful herb for women; it is a soothing, all-round nutritious general tonic.*

sickness, reduces pain in labor and can also be used preventively to help avoid painful menstrual cramps, cystitis and vaginal discharges. It is very beneficial for treating nausea, and is helpful in cases of acute and chronic diarrhea, as well as being a mild and safe helper (particularly in combination with chamomile) for children with stomach complaints. More recently, it has been employed to ward off colds, flu and fever, and as a lotion for treating inflamed skin conditions.

**AVAILABLE FORMS:** The most common form of raspberry available is a tea made from the fresh or dried leaves. It can also be obtained as an extract, and is used in cosmetics and soothing skin lotions. The fruit of the raspberry is also a popular culinary ingredient.

*raspberry leaf*

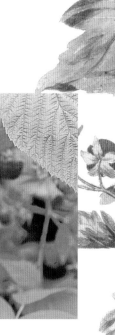

# ROSEHIPS

Dog rose, brier rose, sweet brier
*Rosa canina*
FAMILY: Rosaceae

*"A rose by any other name would smell as sweet," said Juliet. Medicinally, this fragrantly perfumed plant will sweeten your life, health and senses today.*

**DESCRIPTION:** There are more than 12,000 known species of cultivated rose. The common dog rose, a bushy shrub which varies in height from 2–13 feet (0.6–3.9 m), has many stems covered in sharp spines with alternating serrated leaves. It produces its flowers in early summer, with many variations of color from almost white to a very deep pink, and has a delicate, refreshing fragrance. The orange to deep scarlet fruit, known as the hip, is often used medicinally.

*The humble rosehip is a power-packed and potent personal arsenal in the fight against the common cold, the flu and all types of modern-day infections and stresses.*

**HISTORY:** The cultivated rose probably stemmed from northern Persia, spreading across Asia Minor to Greece. The word *rosa* comes from the Greek *rodon*, meaning red — the rose of the ancients was a deep crimson color, provoking the legend of its "having sprung from the blood of Adonis." In the Middle Ages, it became known as canina for its supposed ability to cure mad dog bites or rabies. The ancient Romans used it prolifically, strewing their floors and tables, adding the petals to their wine — roses were a sign of pleasure, the companion to mirth and feasts, but they were also for funerals and adornment to warships. The dog rose has always had the attributes "pleasure mixed with pain." Rose water was prepared by Avicenna in the tenth century, and in the sixteenth century rosehip came into common use as oil of roses.

**MODERN USES:** Rosehips are a valuable vitamin supplement and tonic, containing high levels of vitamins C, A, E, K, P, some B vitamins, iron, copper compounds, and organic acids.

The tea is frequently consumed for colds, flu, allergies, general debility or for just feeling over-tired or stressed. It is also valuable in helping regain strength after any illness. It is often prescribed as a circulatory tonic, for hypertension, infections, indigestion, stomach troubles and as a gargle for sore or bleeding gums or teeth, and mouth ulcers. Rosehips' gentle astringent and cleansing action is also of great help to the liver, gallbladder and kidney systems. The oil may be used to calm and soothe and is generally regarded as bringing peace, so may be helpful for headaches, migraines, muscular tension, premenstrual tension, stress and insomnia. Rose oil is now frequently administered in hospices to bring peace and comfort to the terminally ill.

**AVAILABLE FORMS:** Tea made from its fresh or dried form is the most general use of the rosehip. It is also available as a tincture or extract, or as an oil. Rosehip is an ingredient in many herbal combinations.

*rosehips*

# ROSEMARY

Polar plant, compass weed
*Rosmarinus officinalis*
FAMILY: Labiatae

*"There's rosemary, that's for remembrance," said Ophelia in Shakespeare's* Hamlet.
*Or according to Culpepper, "It quickens a weak memory, and the senses."*

**DESCRIPTION:** This well-known evergreen shrubby herb, native to the Mediterranean coast, has numerous branches with scaly bark, and narrow dark green leathery leaves about 1 inch (2.5 cm) long, with a downy paler underside. The flowers are small, whitish to pale blue; the whole plant is aromatic, due to the high content of volatile oil. The leaves can be gathered throughout the summer, but are at their best while flowering. It has been long known as a medicinal, aromatic, culinary and emotive herb.

**HISTORY:** Ancient lore tells us that rosemary had a reputation for strengthening the memory; hence, it became the emblem of fidelity for lovers. In the Middle Ages, it was used at weddings, funerals and religious ceremonies, and in many magical spells. According to Sir Thomas More, it was the herb "sacred to remembrance, and, therefore, to friendship." Interestingly, it seems to have had this reputation all over the ancient world. In Spain and Italy, particularly, it was considered a safeguard against witches and evil, as they believed it was one of the herbs that gave shelter to the Virgin Mary in her flight to Egypt. Rosemary was used for a vast number of ailments — to purify the air, to prevent infection, to guard against nightmares; it was applied as a remedy for boils, skin afflictions, gout, rheumatism, coughs and fevers; and it was considered an anti-aging remedy, helpful for failing memory, and a boost for general depression.

*Rosemary is a great cleanser, helping to purify the whole body. It is a non-addictive assistant for general lethargy and all those vague symptoms of modern-day life, helping to stimulate the circulation and give your body an all over "spring cleaning."*

62

**MODERN USES:** Rosemary is high in calcium, magnesium, zinc, iron, and vitamins A and C, which may well justify its ancient uses as a memory strengthener and nervine tonic. Nowadays, it is highly regarded as a circulatory stimulant, often indicated for varicose veins, as an antispasmodic, relaxant, carminative, antidepressant and general tonic. It is anti-inflammatory, antiseptic, antifungal, antibacterial, astringent, with anodyne, diuretic and antidepressant properties. It is used to treat many digestive problems such as colic, ulcers, nervous stomach and anorexia, as well as rheumatism, arthritis, gout, menstrual cramps, headaches and migraines; rosemary's bitter elements are of great help in all liver conditions, and to help alleviate hangovers. Externally, rosemary oil is used to treat rheumatism, sciatica, gout, sprains, bruises and neuralgia. It is renowned for its tonic benefits on the skin, the hair and the scalp, is used as an ingredient in soaps, cosmetics, shampoos, and helps stimulate the hair follicles in premature baldness.

**AVAILABLE FORMS:** Fresh leaves and flowers are used as a tea. Rosemary is also available as a tincture, extract or essential oil. It is often found in soap, skin, hair and cosmetic preparations.

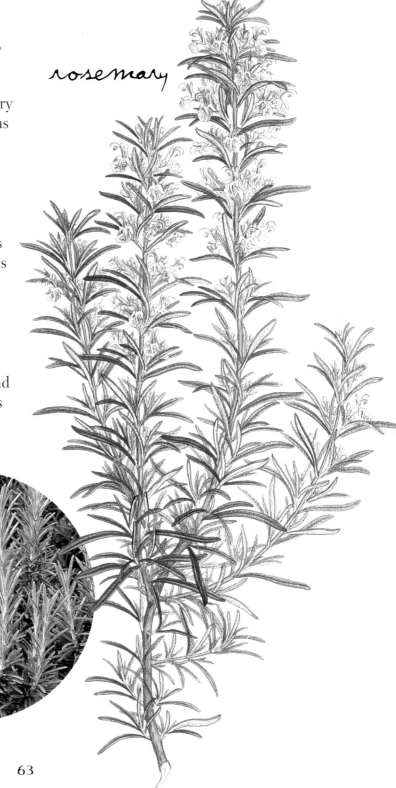

rosemary

# SENNA

Cassia acutifolia, Alexandrian senna, senna pods
*Cassia senna*
FAMILY: Leguminosae

***Senna has been famous for its purgative action since before the ninth century.***

**DESCRIPTION:** This small perennial shrub is about 2 feet (0.6 m) high, with an erect, long-spreading, smooth, pale green stem bearing multiple, divided branches, which have smooth sub-divided leaves, with a faint, peculiar odor, and a sweetish taste. The numerous small yellow flowers are followed by broad oblong fruit pods, which are about 2 inches (5 cm) long, generally each containing about six seeds.

**HISTORY:** Senna is an Arabic name, the drug having been first brought into known medical usage by the physicians of the ninth century in Mecca, the birthplace of Mohammed. It was also extensively cultivated and used medicinally in Africa, India and the Middle East. The early Greeks preferred the pods to the leaves, as they believed they had a less griping effect in their purgative action, the quality for which the herb has become famous across the centuries. It appears the herb was not widely cultivated in England until the early seventeenth century, when it became a common household purgative and laxative, frequently combined with cloves, cinnamon and ginger to help correct nausea and treat many lower bowel conditions, such as chronic constipation and dysentery.

**MODERN USES:** Senna is a purgative, its primary action being on the lower bowel; it increases peristalsis with its action on the intestinal wall; it has a stimulating, slightly griping action. For this reason, it is most often used in combination with other gentler laxatives, such as slippery elm, marshmallow, gentian, ginger and licorice; but be aware, it

*Senna is a powerful purger, always to be used carefully in fresh form. In combination with other gentler herbs, it can be one of the most effective purgatives.*

has a somewhat unpleasant taste to match its actions. It has been used as a liver tonic for bilious disorders associated with constipation, as well as fevers accompanying intestinal infections, but it should not be used for hemorrhoids, colitis or any prolapsed bowel conditions. Taking large doses of the fresh leaf can cause nausea, griping pains and red coloration of the urine. An effective herb, but one to treat with caution.

**AVAILABLE FORMS:** This herb should probably be only used in a prescribed formula — either as extract, tincture, tablet or in combination with other laxative herbal formulas.

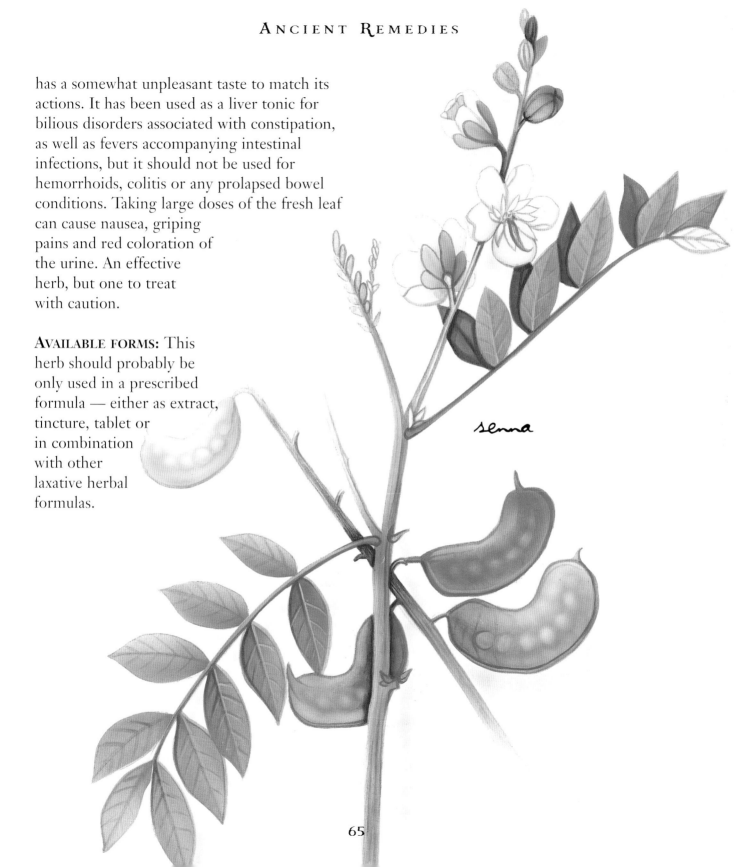

senna

# SLIPPERY ELM

Red elm, moose elm, Indian elm
*Ulmus fulva*
**FAMILY:** Ulmaceae

*Slippery elm bark has many uses, but is particularly beneficial for conditions of the digestive tract, urinary system, the skin and the lungs; it is also a nutritional supplement.*

**DESCRIPTION:** The deciduous slippery elm tree grows to a height of 50 feet (16 m) or more. It has very rough branches, with long, unequally toothed rough leaves, hairy on both sides, with stalkless leaf buds; the inconspicuous flowers are small tufts appearing in clusters in early spring. The pale, whitish, aromatic inner bark is the major medicinal component. Slippery elm is an official drug of the United States Pharmacopoeia.

**HISTORY:** The many forms of elm tree are widely distributed throughout the northern temperate zone; the common elm is a native of Europe, North Africa and Asia Minor; the slippery elm, however, is native to the United States and Canada. Native Americans regarded it as a staple medicine — a tea made from the bark was used as a laxative and treatment for constipation, and an infusion made from the root assisted childbirth and all "internal" problems. In many parts of the world, over the centuries, it was powdered, mixed into a smooth paste with cold water and then added to hot water, milk or fruit juice for treating stomach and intestinal disorders. Its soothing properties were also exercised in the treatments of insomnia, bronchitis, coughs and all types of chest disorders.

**MODERN USES:** In modern times, slippery elm has become recognized as one of the most effective soothers for inflammatory conditions. The powdered root, mixed with water, fruit juice, or mashed with a banana, will assist many irritable bowel conditions, such as colitis, ulcers, stress-related diarrhea, constipation, hemorrhoids and diverticulitis.

*There is no finer food and medicine than this — it is cooling, healing and soothing for the entire digestive tract; it should be a staple supplement in every household.*

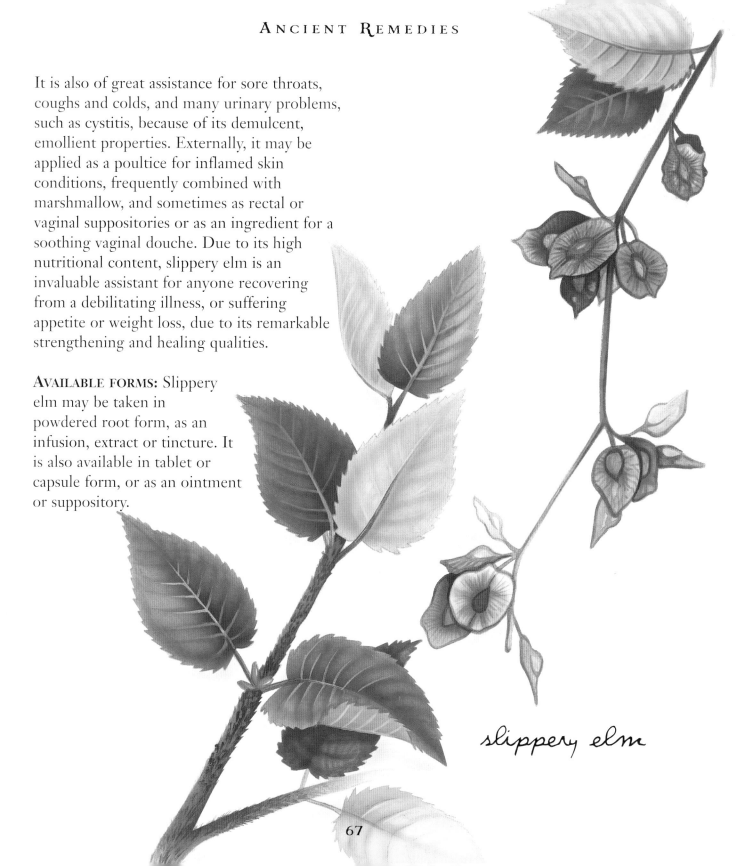

It is also of great assistance for sore throats, coughs and colds, and many urinary problems, such as cystitis, because of its demulcent, emollient properties. Externally, it may be applied as a poultice for inflamed skin conditions, frequently combined with marshmallow, and sometimes as rectal or vaginal suppositories or as an ingredient for a soothing vaginal douche. Due to its high nutritional content, slippery elm is an invaluable assistant for anyone recovering from a debilitating illness, or suffering appetite or weight loss, due to its remarkable strengthening and healing qualities.

**AVAILABLE FORMS:** Slippery elm may be taken in powdered root form, as an infusion, extract or tincture. It is also available in tablet or capsule form, or as an ointment or suppository.

*slippery elm*

# ST. JOHN'S WORT

Hypericum, goatweed, amber, Johnswort
*Hypericum perforatum*
FAMILY: Hypericaceae

*Modern clinical studies reports that true to folklore, St. John's wort is providing enormous relief to people with mild to moderate depression, without the side effects of pharmaceutical antidepressants — a six billion dollar annual worldwide market.*

**DESCRIPTION:** St. John's wort is a perennial plant, rarely more than 3 feet (80 cm) tall, with small, oblong leaves and bright yellow flowers with five petals. The leaves contain numerous oil glands, which are visible as fine, translucent dots when the leaf is held up against the light (hence the specific name, *perforatum*, meaning perforated). The plant is native to Europe, but appears as an introduced weed in Australia and North America.

**HISTORY:** St. John's wort has been valued since antiquity for its healing powers, believed to be derived from St. John the Baptist, as he was beheaded on the day it comes into full flower. Legend has it that the Devil pierced the leaves of the plant with a needle to make it wither, in an attempt to prevent humans from benefiting from its medicinal virtues.

Its Latin name *Hypericum* is derived from the Greek meaning "above pictures," referring to the ancient tradition of placing the plant above shrines to repel evil spirits. In the Middle Ages it was believed that the translucent oil dots, which appear to be fine holes in the leaves, were a sign that the plant was useful in the treatment of wounds from knives and swords — or for treating melancholy, a wounded or pierced heart.

**MODERN USES:** St. John's wort is an excellent wound healing plant. The ruby-red oil produced by steeping the flowers in vegetable oil is particularly useful for this purpose, as well as for various skin complaints. It is also used for the treatment of many forms of neuralgia or nerve damage, bruises, abrasions, rheumatic pain and hemorrhoids.

But what has dramatically shot St. John's wort to fame in the last few years is the fact that it is a powerful herbal antidepressant. Numerous clinical studies have confirmed that St. John's wort extracts are effective in the treatment of mild to severe depression, and some forms of anxiety. Recent research has also indicated that it may be beneficial in treating AIDS, and other studies are starting to indicate that it may have potent antiviral activity, including immunodeficiency conditions.

**AVAILABLE FORMS:** St. John's wort is available as tea, tincture or extract, and as tablets or capsules, or as an oil for topical use. It is also often used in conjunction with other herbs in creams and ointments.

st. john's wort

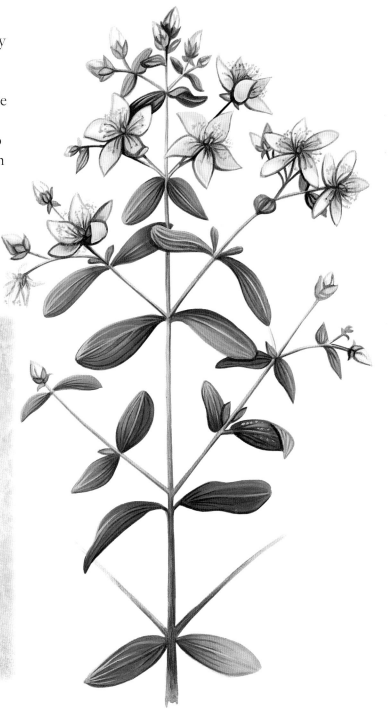

*In Germany, where most of the research on St. John's wort has been conducted, high-strength preparations of the herb have become by far the most popular antidepressant on the market, outselling its nearest competitor by four to one.*

# TEA TREE

Ti tree
*Melaleuca alternifolia*
**FAMILY:** Myrtaceae

*Tea tree is one of the best immune system stimulants you'll find. Remember, though, it's a strong volatile oil — keep it out of the reach of children.*

**DESCRIPTION:** The tea tree is a hardy, medium to tall shrub, native to Australia and New Zealand, growing to about 23 feet (7 m). It is a conifer-like bushy tree, with irregularly arranged, scattered leaves, and a distinctive papery bark. The cream colored or white solitary flower spikes appear in spring or early summer. It grows widely around streams, on swampy flats, and on the coastal and adjacent ranges of eastern Australia.

**HISTORY:** Sir Joseph Banks, the botanist on the *Endeavour*, named the paperbark trees around Botany Bay "tea trees," as he thought the fine, almost weeping leaves may have provided a substitute for the real brew. Well, he was wrong; however, the Aborigines had it right, they'd been using it for eons as a medicinal herb for many of their general health problems. At the beginning of the twentieth century, Australian scientists discovered its benefits as an antiseptic and healing agent, particularly for open wounds, infections and gangrene, and the oil received widespread recognition during World War II, when it was found that its highly antiseptic, antiviral and antibacterial powers were much more powerful than the available pharmaceutical drugs.

**MODERN USES:** Tea tree is one of the only essential oils known to be antiseptic, antifungal, antiviral and antibacterial. It has gained widespread medicinal use for a whole array of modern-day conditions, especially acne, dry itchy skin, dermatitis, bruises, burns

*Tea tree is a great natural cure-all — keep tea tree oil in the medicine cabinet to use as a handy antiseptic and antifungal agent. It's also great in vaporizers to relieve sniffles.*

and insect bites. One of tea tree's most beneficial external uses is as an antiseptic for wounds or cuts, or as an antifungal agent for athlete's foot (tinea), ringworm and vaginal yeast infections. Tea tree is an immunostimulant, and so is used internally to help boost the immune system against infections, colds, flu and most sinus and respiratory tract conditions. The oil is very effectively employed externally for muscular pain, varicose veins and hemorrhoids, and is also used for mouth ulcers, cold sores, herpes, abscesses, dandruff and scalp conditions. Tea tree is also used as an adjunct in ridding the body of unwanted vermin such as lice, ticks and leeches.

**AVAILABLE FORMS:** Most commonly found as an oil, tea tree extract is also found in cosmetic preparations such as shampoos, moisturizers, creams and veterinary preparations.

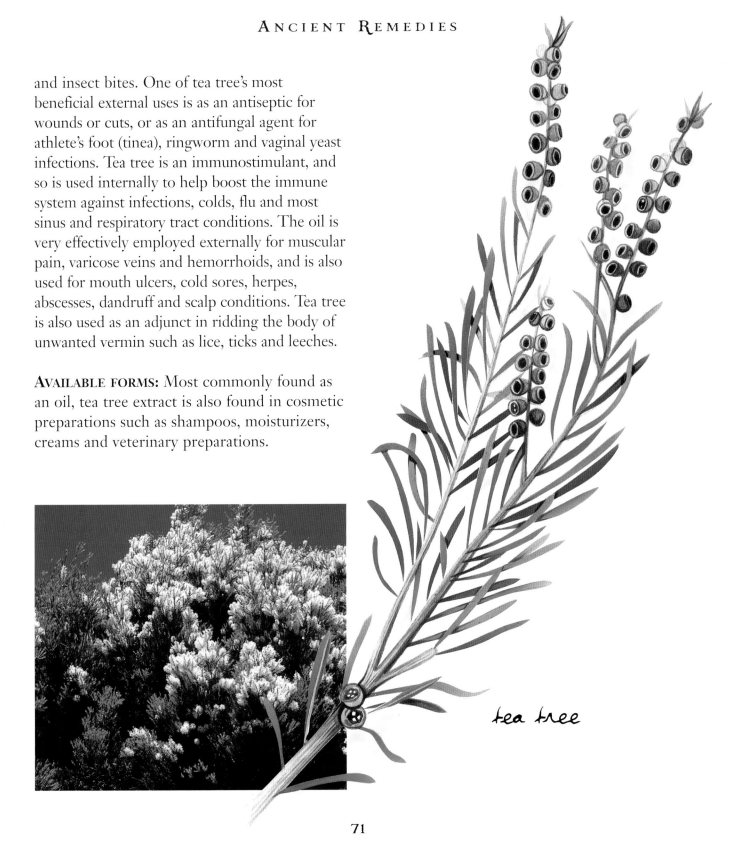

tea tree

# THYME

Common thyme, garden thyme
*Thymus vulgaris*
**FAMILY:** Labiatae

*We should all make time for this mighty little action-packed herb,*
*ever ready to help you escape the ravages of time.*

**DESCRIPTION:** The common thyme is a perennial plant with a woody, fibrous root and numerous hard, round, branched stems, usually from 4–8 inches (10–20 cm) high. It has small greenish gray leaves and its white to lilac flowers appear in early summer to late fall (autumn). Its seeds are round and very small — there are about 170,000 to the ounce — and they retain their germinating power for three years. The whole plant has a pleasant aromatic odor and a spicy taste.

**HISTORY:** The herb's name possibly came from the Greek word "to fumigate," as it was utilized as a cleanser, or from their word denoting "courage," the plant being held in ancient times as a great source of invigoration and strength. It was used by the ancient Egyptians for their embalming processes and as a symbol of bravery. The Arabs have honored it since ancient times as a medicine for digestive disorders. The herb's volatile essential oil, thymol, was first isolated in Germany in the early eighteenth century, and has been used in many pharmaceutical preparations since then for its antiseptic,

astringent, tonic, and carminative features. In the sixteenth century, European herbalists recommended it for "wambling and gripings of the belly," for rheumatism, headache and drowsiness, and, according to Culpepper, "a certain remedy for that troublesome complaint, the night-mare."

**MODERN USES:** Thyme has a power-packed antiseptic action — it will go in fighting for you against sore throats, catarrh, colds, coughs, flu, fevers and most infections. Modern studies have shown it to be a powerful aid in alleviating certain types of nerve pain, such as sciatica, menstrual cramps and general debility. Thyme also has a strong effective action on the digestive system, especially for stimulating the appetite, for indigestion, stomach ulcers, diarrhea or constipation. It can also act as a cleansing liver tonic and its tonic action on the nervous system makes it a useful assistant for relieving exhaustion, tension and anxiety. Externally, it can be applied to stimulate circulation, for rheumatism, for cuts and wounds, and for many skin conditions including shingles and herpes; it is used as a strengthening tonic for the scalp to prevent or stop hair loss. It can also be taken internally as a vermifuge — an ingredient in combinations for expelling worms and other parasites from the intestines. Be a little careful with internal use, as excessive doses of the oil can overstimulate the thyroid gland and cause some unwanted hormonal problems.

**AVAILABLE FORMS:** Apart from using the leaves of the fresh herb in cooking, an infusion, oil, tincture or extract are the most common ways of benefiting from thyme. It is also used as a cosmetic and aromatherapy agent.

*thyme*

*Thyme is the chief ingredient of most modern mouthwashes, and is a common ingredient in many gargles and toothpastes. Try it fresh to get rid of bad breath.*

# VALERIAN

All-heal, great wild valerian, fragrant valerian, phu
*Valeriana officinalis*
FAMILY: Valerianaceae

*Valerian is the modern-day tranquilizer, allaying pain, calming the nerves, and promoting refreshing sleep, without the hangover or addictive side effects of pharmaceutical drugs.*

**DESCRIPTION:** Valerian is native to Europe and western Asia, and is now found in most parts of the temperate world. It is a perennial plant, growing about 2–4 feet (0.6–1.2 m) high, with one round hairy stem growing from the root (the part used in medicines), terminating in two or more pairs of flowering stems, with alternately paired rich, dark green serrated leaves. The masses of small whitish pink to reddish flowers have a fragrant smell, although the plant and root are considered to have a strong, unpleasant odor.

**HISTORY:** The first recorded mention of valerian seems to have been around the ninth or tenth century, when Arab physicians used a decoction for cramp, restlessness and fevers. It was referred to in the medical records of Gaelan and Dioscorides as Phu, or Fu, relating to its offensive odor; its name probably derives from the Latin *valere*, meaning to be in health.

Valerian has always been used for its sedative, carminative and antispasmodic properties. It was known to the Anglo-Saxons, who ate it as a salad and to ward off the plague. It was particularly used in Britain in the Middle Ages for conditions such as hysteria, insomnia, St. Vitus' Dance, neuralgic pain, general debility, croup, coughs, palpitations, breathlessness and dizziness. Valerian was also commonly prescribed to treat shell-shocked soldiers and stressed civilians in both world wars.

**MODERN USES:** Valerian is still widely used as a carminative, anti-spasmodic and nerve tonic; its chemical formulation was the basis for pharmaceutical antidepressants; however, when used in its natural form, it does not have the side effects or addictive characteristics of the synthetic drug. Valerian helps allay pain, and assists in depression, stress, insomnia, and anxiety.

Due to its antispasmodic action, valerian is also effective in treating painful menstrual cramps, stomach cramps, migraines, rheumatic pain and neuralgia. It is being more frequently used for circulatory conditions and, in combination with other herbs, for treating hypertension and palpitations. Large doses, however, should be avoided, as they can cause headaches or stupor. Externally, it has been used as a wash for sores and acne. In the garden, valerian is an instant attraction for cats (and for rats — it has been said the Pied Piper attained fame with the valerian roots secreted around his person).

**AVAILABLE FORMS:** The rootstock can be taken as tea, infusion, tincture or extract. This herb is also available in many sedative herbal compounds, or as tablets and capsules. All preparations may be obtained from your health food store.

*Culpepper tells us "It is under the influence of Mercury and therefore has a warming facility."*

*Valerian is primarily a quieting, soothing natural tranquilizer, Nature's own gentle, antistress agent.*

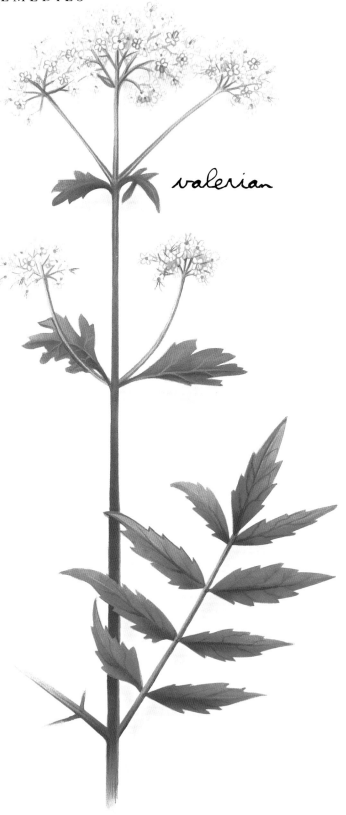

valerian

# WILLOW BARK

White willow, European willow
*Salix alba*
**FAMILY:** Salicaceae

*Willow is the natural source of salicin, later to become synthesized as aspirin. It has been used to help pain, fever and rheumatism for over two thousand years.*

**DESCRIPTION:** A large, deciduous tree growing up to 75 feet (25 m) high, the white willow is found in damp, moist places in north Africa, central Asia and Europe, from where it was introduced to northeastern America and other parts of the world. It has a rough, grayish bark, easily separable from the tree in summer, and its alternate, serrated leaves are ash gray, and silky on both sides. The male and female flowers occur on separate trees.

**HISTORY:** The ability of willow bark to ease the pain of joint conditions, rheumatism and general aches and pains has been known since the times of the ancient Greeks. Throughout the Middle Ages, it was highly regarded for reducing any form of inflammation, particularly used for all rheumatic or gouty conditions or conditions considered to be brought on by the damp or moist, a reflection of its place of growth. The bark was also used to treat fevers, agues and plagues, and the many common digestive disorders, such as dyspepsia, flatulence, diarrhea and dysentery. Its astringent properties enabled it to be used for gum or teeth troubles and sore throats, and externally for sores, bleeding, burns and wounds.

**MODERN USES:** Willow contains salicin, a compound which converts to salicylic acid in the body, and is closely related to aspirin, the synthetic drug formulated in more recent times. Medicinally, it is a painkiller, antiseptic, astringent, diuretic, febrifuge and tonic.

Willow bark is still particularly indicated for cases of rheumatoid or arthritic pain, gout,

*Willow bark is one of the best natural painkillers around, gentle on the stomach and without unpleasant side effects on the kidneys or liver.*

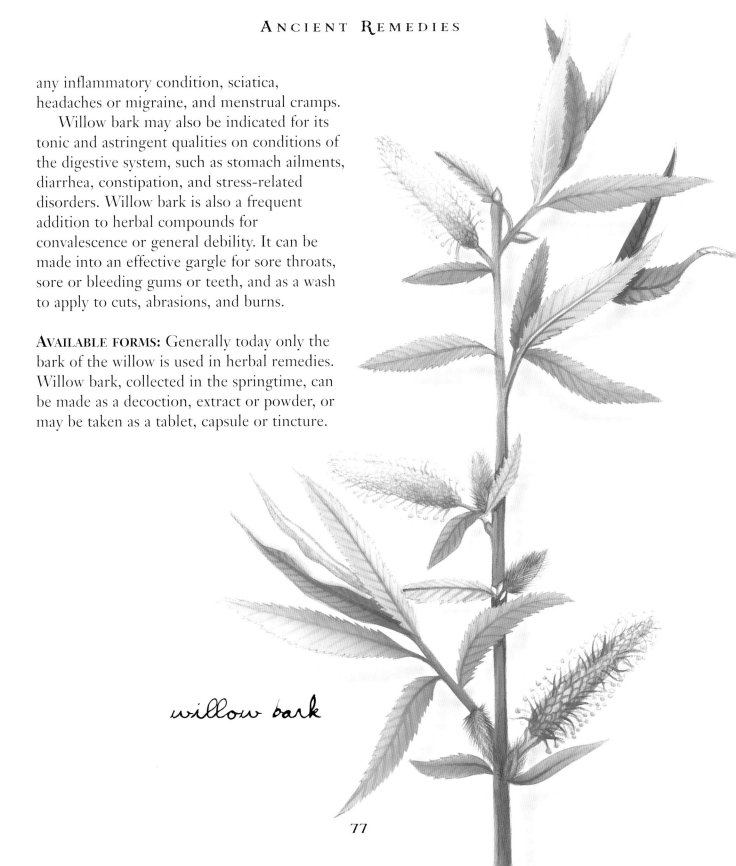

any inflammatory condition, sciatica, headaches or migraine, and menstrual cramps.

Willow bark may also be indicated for its tonic and astringent qualities on conditions of the digestive system, such as stomach ailments, diarrhea, constipation, and stress-related disorders. Willow bark is also a frequent addition to herbal compounds for convalescence or general debility. It can be made into an effective gargle for sore throats, sore or bleeding gums or teeth, and as a wash to apply to cuts, abrasions, and burns.

**AVAILABLE FORMS:** Generally today only the bark of the willow is used in herbal remedies. Willow bark, collected in the springtime, can be made as a decoction, extract or powder, or may be taken as a tablet, capsule or tincture.

*willow bark*

# WITCH HAZEL

Spotted alder, winterbloom, snapping hazelnut
*Hamamelis virginiana*
FAMILY: Hamamelidaceae

*If you need to stop bleeding in a hurry, try witch hazel.*
*Due to high levels of tannins in the plants it has an astringent effect which*
*makes it a remedy for cuts and wounds.*

**DESCRIPTION:** Witch hazel is a deciduous shrub or small tree, growing to about 10–12 feet (3–3.6 m) in height, a native of the United States and Canada. It has branching, crooked stems and small, smooth, downy, grayish leaves. The narrow, yellow, ribbon-like petals grow in clusters and bloom in fall (autumn) when the leaves are falling. The seed is seldom produced except in its native habitat — the seeds are ejected violently when ripe, hence its name snapping hazelnut.

*Witch hazel will tone up your life —*

*its astringent, tonic and yet relaxing*

*qualities can help you through all sorts*

*of modern-day emergencies, without*

*resorting to drugs.*

**HISTORY:** The name *hamamelis* comes from the Greek words "apple" and "together," since the flowers and fruit of the tree, which resembles an apple tree, are produced at the same time. Forked witch hazel branches were long employed as water-divining rods by Native Americans, who brought the plant's medicinal virtues to the attention of the European settlers. The Native Americans mainly used the leaves and bark as poultices for painful swellings, skin conditions, bruises, or as a tea for diarrhea, internal bleeding, nose bleeds, hemorrhoids, or to stop any sort of wound bleeding. After its introduction to Europe, it became widely used as a general household remedy for burns, insect bites, skin conditions, hemorrhoids and varicose veins.

**MODERN USES:** Witch hazel is still highly regarded for its strong astringent, tonic and slightly sedative properties, and for its ability to stop bleeding. Internally, it may be added to herbal compounds to assist bowel conditions, such as diarrhea, ulcers, varicose veins and hemorrhoids. It is frequently prescribed for problems with excessive menstruation, excessive mucus discharges (resulting from infection or chronic conditions such as colds, allergies and sinusitis) and as an aid in helping the body recover from any debilitating illness. It may also be used as an ingredient in douches or pessaries for vaginitis, thrush, or hemorrhoids. Externally, it is most effective in treating bruises and sprains, cuts, bites and stings, minor burns and any inflammatory skin conditions. In a diluted form, witch hazel is helpful for treating eye inflammations and is added to many cosmetics for its tonic and soothing properties.

**AVAILABLE FORMS:** Witch hazel may be purchased at your health food store as a decoction, extract, tincture or tea, but it is most commonly found in distilled liquid form as an ingredient in herbal compounds, in cream, lotion or ointment form, and as a cosmetic additive.

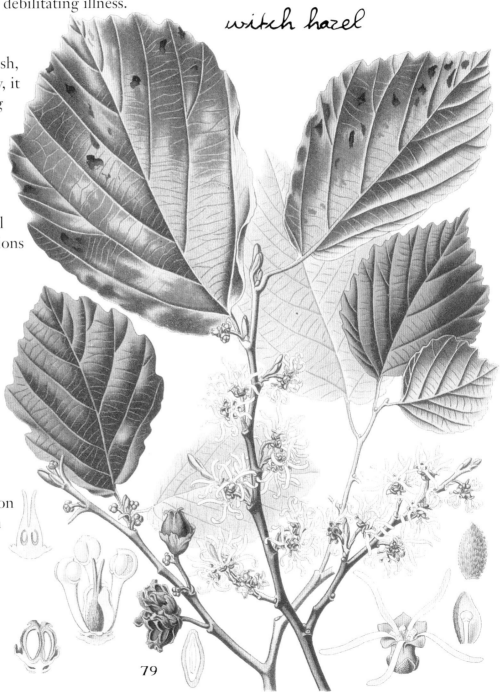

witch hazel

# YARROW

Milfoil, soldier's woundwort, staunchgrass, sneezewort, kiss-me-quick
*Achillea millefolium*
FAMILY: Compositae

*"Out, damned spot!"*
*If Lady Macbeth had had some yarrow around to stem the flow*
*of blood, things might have been a bit neater —*
*but then, we may not have had such a good story.*

**DESCRIPTION:** Yarrow is a prolific, aromatic, perennial plant, common all over the temperate world, with flowering stems, 1–2 feet (30–60 cm) high. The Latin name *milfoil*, meaning thousand leaves, comes from the finely-divided alternating feathery leaves. The many dense heads form five or six florets of white or pinkish flowers, similar to miniature daisies and grouped in tight, flat clusters, with yellow or brown centred disks; the whole plant has white, silky hairs.

**HISTORY:** Yarrow is known in British history as the soldier's herb, or *Herba Militaris*, recognized since ancient times for its ability to stem the flow of blood. The Latin name reputedly comes from Achilles, who had his wounds dressed at the siege of Troy by a weeping Aphrodite to stop the bleeding and ease the pain. In many cultures, it has long been used to ease or heal wounds, particularly wounds of war and battle.

In Anglo-Saxon times, the Druids used it as a "magickal" herb of great power — both to

*Growing this pretty, feathery plant in your garden will do wonders for your "instant" emergency medical kit. Keep it on hand for the first sign of a cold.*

protect against evil, and also, when called for, to invoke the blackest magic.

European gypsies called it "the carpenter's herb," because it was always at hand when any workman's tools slipped. It has also been used for thousands of years by the Chinese for divination — dried yarrow stems were used to see the future with the divinatory *I Ching*, the Chinese Book of Changes.

**MODERN USES:** The whole plant is used apart from the roots; today, it is recognized as a diaphoretic, astringent, antiseptic, tonic and stimulant. Its most common uses are still as a wound healer — to stop bleeding — and for general body system cleansing and for treating colds, flu and fever. It has a beneficial effect on circulation and so is extremely useful for conditions such as high blood pressure, kidney disorders, hemorrhoids, digestive disorders, constipation, varicose veins, menstrual troubles, psoriasis and many other skin conditions.

The fresh leaf is used for toothache or abscesses as a compress, or rolled and placed into the nose to stop nosebleeds, or placed directly onto a small cut to stop bleeding.

**AVAILABLE FORMS:** Available as fresh leaf tea, fresh plant infusion, ointment or cream, cosmetic or tincture or extract form.

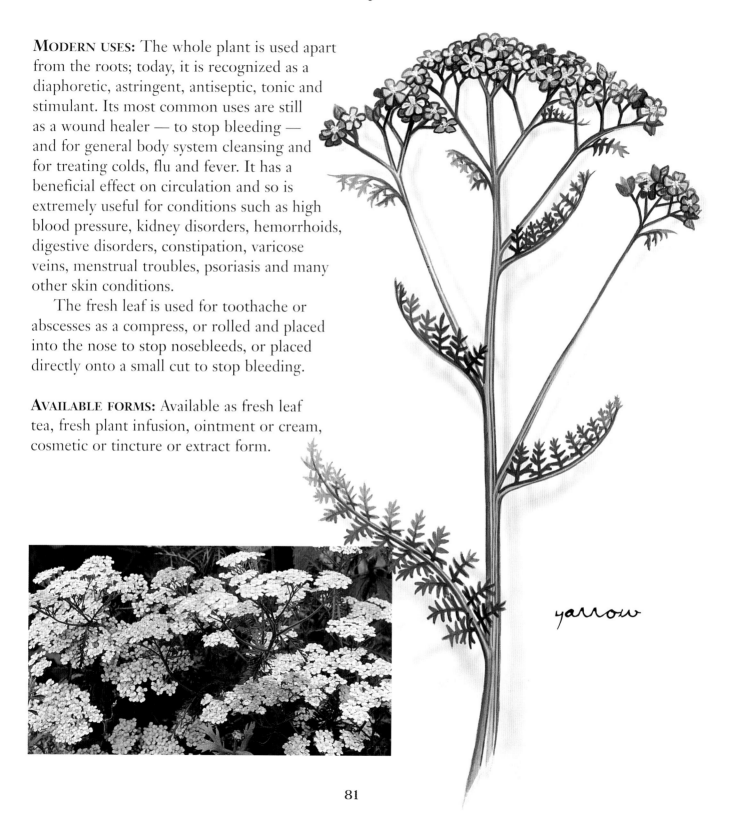

yarrow

# OTHER ANCIENT REMEDIES FOR MODERN AILMENTS

People around the world are starting to realize that ancient remedies can play an important part in our lives. More and more, we are looking at our illnesses in a holistic way — not just trying to treat separate symptoms. When we feel unwell, we look at where we went wrong and what we can do about it.

Modern-day living has brought us increased stress, a range of dietary disorders, a high level of pollutants in the world around us, increased drug use, and growing depression. It is said that we are what we think. Today, it appears, many of us don't think well of ourselves, and in general, we're not well. However, many of us are now starting to investigate the ways in which we can experience good health, rather than just limiting ourselves to treating diseases. There is a growing understanding that the choices are ours and that our choices are greater when we refer to the knowledge of the past and adapt it to our "fast-pace" way of life.

Ancient wisdom tells us that "change is the only truth in the Universe." Let's experience, feel, grow and manifest, and make ourselves a part of it all. We can make our own change and choose health. If we listen to those whispers, ancient wisdom will become part of our modern life.

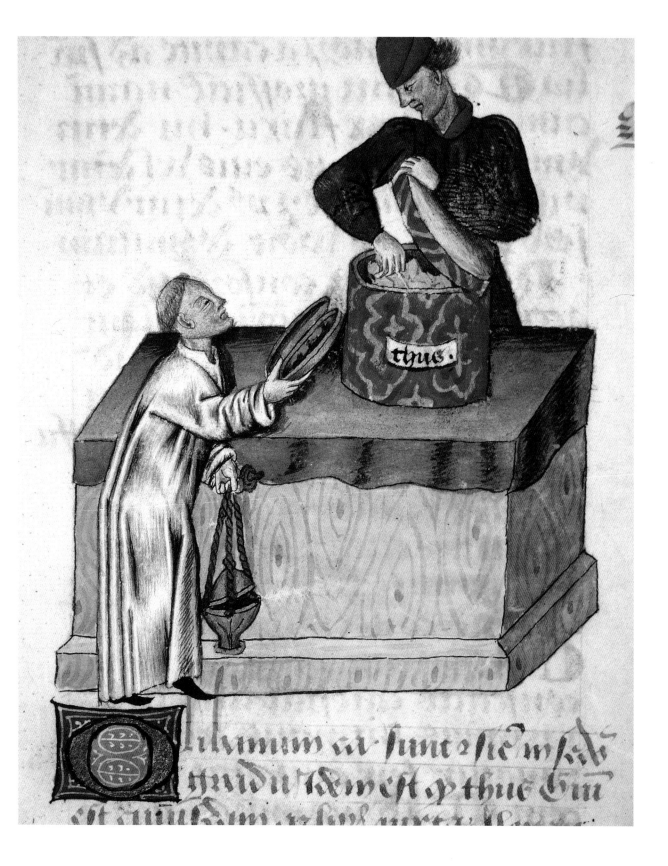

thus.

*World Health Organization statistics*

*show that the levels of heart disease*

*in southern Europe are lower than those*

*in northern Europe. It seems that the*

*Mediterranean diet — which is high in*

*salads, fish, rice, fruit and red wine —*

*and perhaps the more relaxed pace of life,*

*the hot weather, and a broader network*

*of family and friends, may provide*

*protection from heart disease.*

*Interestingly, the incidence of heart*

*disease is particularly high in Scotland*

*and Northern Ireland.*

## FOOD AND NUTRITION

Much has been written about the importance of a good diet and a healthy lifestyle, and yet today we seem to have a wide range of health problems associated with eating. Disorders such as anorexia and bulimia are increasing, and many in the West are overweight.

Like your car, your body needs fuel. Almost three-quarters of the energy (or kilojoules) you consume is used to keep your organs functioning, renew your cells, circulate your blood and keep your body temperature normal. Only when your intake of energy is more than your body requires will the excess be stored as fat.

The food we eat comprises six basic groups: carbohydrates, fiber, vitamins, minerals, proteins and fats. The aim is to maintain a balance that suits you. In general, it is best to eat a diet which is high in fiber, fresh fruit and vegetables, and low in fat, salt, sugar and highly processed foods.

Protein foods, such as poultry, fish, lean meats, nuts, cheese, yogurt and eggs, should form only a small part of your diet, as too much fat, saturated animal fat in particular, has been linked to higher incidence of heart disease.

One of our main requirements is water, given that about 70 percent of our body is water. It is needed to form the blood and body fluids which maintain the body's temperature, carry the essential nutrients all round the body and help remove waste products. You should try to have six or eight glasses of pure water a day, or have a generous intake of fruits and foods high in water, to help keep your system running well.

Most important, work out a diet and exercise regime that suits you. Metabolisms differ from person to person and we all have differing nutrient requirements, so find out how you can best meet your own needs. It is important to find the right balance for you.

## AROMATHERAPY

Aromatherapy is a major modern-day revival of an ancient healing art. No one knows exactly where and when aromatherapy began, but the medicinal use of plant oils is recorded in some of the earliest hinese medical documents, from around 4,000 years ago, as well as in ancient Egyptian, Greek and European history. The ancient Persians also revered flower waters, which they distilled from roses, orange blossom and herbs, and used for cosmetics and as remedies for sickness. In the eleventh century the Persian philosopher and physician Avicenna refined the distillation process and introduced purer essential oils. The first recorded use of plant oils in Britain seems to have been in the thirteenth century. From this time on they were widely used in much of Europe as perfumes, antiseptics and medicines. The early twentieth century saw a revival of interest in natural treatments and an increasing demand for pure plant oils.

Essential oils can be used to enhance every aspect of health and well-being. They are used in many ways, such as in atomizers, in baths, foot baths, sitz baths, compresses, inhalations, oil burners, vaporizers and as massage oils. In some cases, such as rosemary and lavender, they can be applied directly to the temples and neck to relieve headache and stress.

Research has been done to estimate the levels of stress people, on average, experience when coping with change in their lives. On a scale of 100, the death of a spouse or loved one rates 100, getting divorced rates 75, moving house rates 65, being fired rates 47, trouble at work rates 23, a change in sleeping habits rates 16, and so on.

Essential oils, with their gentle therapeutic properties, can help us when we are coping with life's pressures. They can relax or stimulate the physical, nervous, emotional and energy systems, thus helping to restore balance in our more stressful times.

Aromatherapy is free from side-effects and suitable for people of all ages, even babies. It is thought to be particularly helpful in treating chronic and recurring conditions.

Practitioners claim that a wide range of illnesses can be treated successfully and that there is often almost immediate improvement when treating nervous conditions (particularly depression, anxiety and stress-induced disorders), insomnia, pain, arthritis and skin problems.

## THE ESSENTIAL OILS

| NAME | PROPERTIES | CAUTION |
| --- | --- | --- |
| **Basil**<br>*Ocimum basilicum* | Digestive • respiratory • soothing • calming • relaxing to muscles • head-clearing • uplifting • clarifying • aphrodisiac • mentally stimulating • refreshing • aid to concentration • useful for soothing skin abrasions | Avoid use during pregnancy |
| **Chamomile**<br>*Matricaria chamomilla (German), Anthemis nobilis (Roman)* | Soothing • mildly antiseptic • analgesic • calming • relaxing to muscles • digestive • balancing for the female system • refreshing • anti-inflammatory • treatment for skin, hair and scalp • treatment for insomnia • mild anaesthetic | Should not be used in the early months of pregnancy |
| **Cedarwood**<br>*Juniper virginiana* | Antiseptic • digestive • astringent • skin toning • calming • aphrodisiac • harmonizing • strengthening • sedative • soothing • diuretic | Avoid use during pregnancy |
| **Cinnamon**<br>*Cinnamomum zeylanicum* | Antiseptic • digestive • respiratory • toning for skin • aphrodisiac • hemostatic • astringent • warming and soothing to skin • uplifting | Avoid use during pregnancy |
| **Clary sage**<br>*Salvia sclarea* | Soothing • anti-inflammatory • calming • astringent • tonifying • warming • relaxing • uplifting • euphoria-producing • balancing female system • antidepressant | Avoid use during pregnancy, if you have high blood pressure or after alcohol |
| **Cypress**<br>*Cupressus sempervirens* | Balancing to the female system • stimulating • circulatory • respiratory • decongestive • head-clearing • antispasmodic • gently diuretic • refreshing • relaxing • astringent • treatment for skin • deodorizing | Avoid use if you have high blood pressure and during pregnancy |
| **Eucalytpus**<br>*Eucalyptus globulus* | Head-clearing • refreshing • stimulating • uplifting • invigorating • respiratory • decongestive • antiseptic • cooling • cleansing • anti-inflammatory • antispasmodic • analgesic | Avoid use if you have high blood pressure or are an epileptic |
| **Frankincense**<br>*Boswellia thurifera* | Nervine • respiratory • restorative • beneficial to the female system • rejuvenating • comforting • relaxing • soothing • fear-dispelling | |
| **Geranium**<br>*Pelargonium graveolens* | Antiseptic • antidepressant • anti-inflammatory • diuretic • balancing • tonifying • warming • refreshing • relaxing • harmonizing • treatment for skin | |
| **Jasmine**<br>*Jasminum grandiflorum* | Relaxing • uplifting • beneficial to the female system • aphrodisiac • strong sensual stimulant • soothing • confidence-building • antidepressant • fear-dispelling • skin-softening | Avoid use during pregnancy |

# THE ESSENTIAL OILS

| NAME | PROPERTIES | CAUTION |
|---|---|---|
| **Lavender**<br>*Lavandula officinalis* | Head-clearing • respiratory • skin-healing • nervine • relaxing to muscles • digestive • sedative • calming • balancing to emotions • analgesic • antiseptic • antibacterial • decongestive • antidepressant • refreshing • relaxing • soothing | |
| **Lemon**<br>*Citrus limomum* | Antiseptic • physically stimulating • skin tonic • antibacterial • astringent • diuretic • circulatory • refreshing • cooling • uplifting • stimulating • motivating • deodorizing | Phototoxic — do not use on the skin in sunlight |
| **Marjoram**<br>*Origanum majorana* | Antispasmodic • carminative • respiratory • nervine • calming • relaxing to muscles • digestive • sedative • warming • fortifying | Avoid use during pregnancy |
| **Orange**<br>*Citrus aurantium* | Relaxing • astringent • refreshing • uplifting • antidepressant | |
| **Peppermint**<br>*Mentha piperita* | Digestive • carminative • respiratory • anti-inflammatory • balancing to the female system • cooling (and warming) • clearing • relaxing to muscles • refreshing | Avoid use during pregnancy |
| **Rose**<br>*Rosa damascena (rose otto), Rosa centifolia (rose absolute)* | Antibacterial • balancing • astringent • antiseptic • antidepressant • anti-inflammatory • aphrodisiac • digestive • relaxing • soothing • sensual • confidence-building • beneficial to female system | |
| **Rosemary**<br>*Rosemarinus officinalis* | Invigorating • digestive • nervine • respiratory • circulatory • muscular • uplifting • stimulating • refreshing • clarifying • treatment for skin, hair and scalp • memory-enhancing | Avoid use if you have high blood pressure, during pregnancy or if you are an epileptic. |
| **Sage**<br>*Salvia officinalis* | Diuretic • analgesic • antiseptic • nervine • relaxing • decongestant • refreshing • appetite stimulant • healing to skin • deodorant and antiperspirant • astringent • stimulating | Avoid use during pregnancy |
| **Sandalwood**<br>*Santalum album* | Digestive • calming • relaxing • soothing • softening and healing to skin • antispasmodic • antidepressant • sedative • warming • confidence-building • grounding | |
| **Tea tree**<br>*Melaleuca alternifolia* | Antiseptic • antifungal • digestive • healing to skin • antibacterial • respiratory • decongestive • strengthening to the immune system • insect repellent | |
| **Thyme**<br>*Thymus vulgaris* | Antiseptic • disinfectant • circulatory • stimulating • respiratory • nervine • cleansing and toning to skin, hair and scalp • relaxing to muscles • refreshing • strengthens the immune system • fortifying | Avoid use during pregnancy |

## TRADITIONAL CHINESE MEDICINE

While the Egyptian pharaohs were having pyramids built, the ancient Chinese emperors were obsessed with medicine. The Chinese herbal tradition dates back about 4,000 years. Taoist legend claims that the so-called father of traditional Chinese medicine, Shen Nung (2000 B.C.) is said to have introduced the concept of yin and yang, the two fundamental principles of the universe — the feminine, passive and yielding; and the masculine, active and assertive — after his enlightenment from the god Pan Ku.

The basic theory behind traditional Chinese medicine is to relate the duality of yin and yang with the life force or chi, and balance them within the body.

Illness was believed to result from an imbalance between yin and yang and the body's chi, and death intervened when they ceased to flow in harmony.

Over the centuries, traditional Chinese medicine maintained its strength and power at a grassroots level. The "barefoot doctors" were skilled at administering the ancient herbal prescriptions for all the common country ailments.

Today, Chinese herbal medicine is considered an orthodox therapy, having overcome the hurdle of the twentieth century scientific revolution and its effectiveness has resulted in its being investigated and accepted all over the world

Diagnosis is made by analyzing the individual's response to the five elements: fire, water, earth, metal and wood. These elements relate to the body's organs and their ability to deal with both their genetic inheritance and external forces. All energy and illness relate back to the elements, so by treating deficiencies in the elements, yin/yang harmony is restored and the disease reversed. As in most traditional medical practices, the principle is that a weak organism will succumb to disease.

The philosophy behind traditional Chinese medicine is that the causes of illness are emotions such as excess joy or sadness, anger, depression, obsessiveness, worry, grief and fear. These emotions can cause a breakdown in the body's defence mechanisms and lead to ill health.

The principle is that each negative pattern or emotion affects a certain part of the body. Each organ has a specific target emotion; for example, fear affects the kidneys, anger affects the liver, depression affects the lungs. Taking the diagnostic pulses shows the practitioner which organs, and therefore which emotions, need to be targeted. Once targeted, the practitioner will generally prescribe an "individually designed" formula which may contain herbal, mineral and sometimes animal ingredients.

Chinese herbalism has been shown to help almost any ailment, and it is backed by thousands of years of research. It is particularly effective in the treatment of conditions such as allergies, arthritis, skin infections, migraines and digestive disorders.

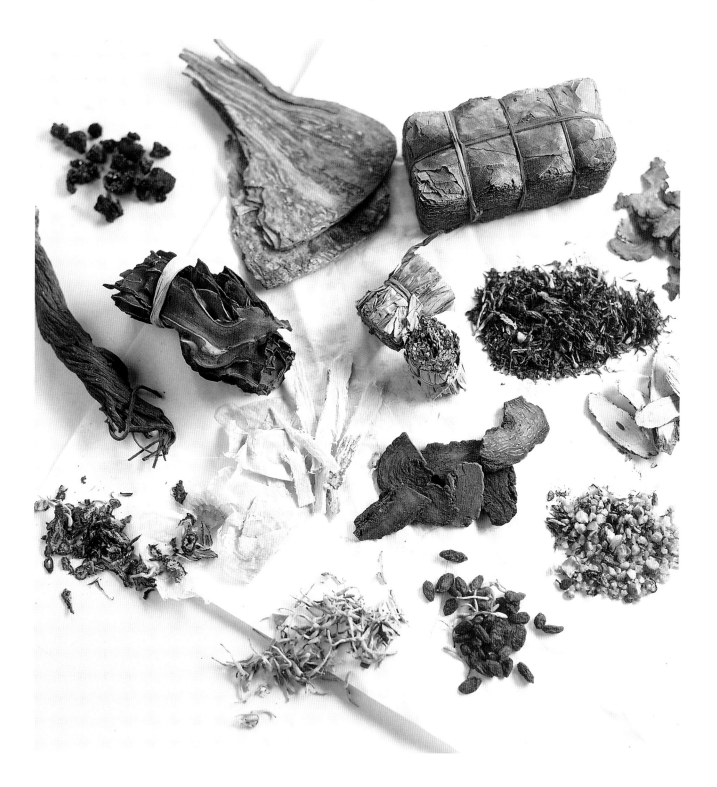

## MASSAGE

The soothing, relaxing power of touch is a great healer. From the time we are born, we crave touch. We need the closeness it provides and the reassurance of physical contact. Of all the healing arts, massage is probably one of the oldest and simplest. Historical artifacts show that the Chinese were using massage techniques as early as 3000 B.C. and the Indian Ayurvedic doctors around 1800 B.C.

Hippocrates, considered the father of western medicine, wrote in the fourth century B.C. that "the physician must be experienced in many things, but assuredly in rubbing ... for rubbing can bind a joint that is loose and loosen a joint that is too rigid." Julius Caesar, an epileptic, was daily pinched all over to relieve recurring headaches and neuralgia. Pliny, the renowned Roman naturalist and healer, regularly received a "rub" to alleviate chronic asthma.

In modern times, massage has become recognized as an essential aid to the physical treatment of stress-related conditions. We use it instinctively when we stroke our children, rub our temples when we're tired, or when we go to a practitioner to ease sore back and neck muscles.

The physical benefits of massage, when combined with the psychological benefits of the underlying warmth, reassurance and trust, can provide a powerful sense of well-being.

The most common and effective use of massage is to relax the body and mind, and so relieve the strains and tensions of daily life.

Physically, it improves blood circulation, tones the muscular and nervous systems, and helps the body assimilate food and eliminate waste products and toxins. On a psychological and emotional level, its calming and soothing effects can help everyone deal with the strains and tensions of daily life, and assist with the treatment of most health disorders.

There are many different types of massage, from the general Swedish relaxation massage to the specific therapeutic variations, such as remedial, shiatsu, deep tissue, kinesiology, lymphatic drainage, Rolfing and sports massage.

## CLEANSING TECHNIQUES

Nature tells us we need to sleep at night and when we're sick in order to restore our energy levels. We all need to rest at some time and, in the same way, it's important to allow the hard-working organs of our body to rest by going on a cleansing diet. Folk practitioners through the ages have urged that eating little during illness aids the body's natural curative function, provided it is done wisely.

Despite our great medical progress in the twentieth century, our view of disease differs little from ancient concepts. It's just that for us "evil germs" have replaced the "evil spirits" of the ancients. We believe that germs go around and diseases are caught, and it is circumstances beyond our control that make us sick. Yet it is probably our weakened resistance to conditions that allows germs to take hold.

Allowing our system to rest helps it build the strength necessary to fight off the unwelcome little visitors that attack our immune system. Throughout history, "rest cures" have involved fasting, cleansing and special diets that are designed to restore the body's equilibrium and eliminate accumulated toxins and wastes.

While going through a cleansing process, the eliminative organs of the body (the kidneys, liver, lungs, intestines and skin) may become overloaded, which can cause a temporary worsening of any condition, or some unpleasant and unwelcome symptoms such as headaches, diarrhea, catarrh and fever. This is called a "healing crisis" and is part of the body's process of regaining its vitality. Be careful, however, and if unexpected things start happening, check with your health practitioner.

If you have a serious medical condition, it is important to undertake a cleansing diet only under the guidance of your practitioner. Never stop taking prescribed medication without checking with your doctor.

There are many sorts of cleansing techniques available. Some of these include juices (fruit and vegetable only, raw food or special diets (such as macrobiotic, vegetarian or vegan), external cleansing (such as saunas, spas, steam baths), regular aromatherapy and lymphatic treatment, and even visualization and meditation.

As with any dramatic change of lifestyle, fasting should be monitored carefully; always make sure sufficient fluids are taken when fasting. An example of a simple seven-day cleansing diet, which will help invigorate your whole system is adjacent.

## A Simple, Seven-Day Cleansing Diet

*Check with your doctor before commencing any diet or exercise program.*

For two or three days prior to commencing this diet, eat only raw vegetables, a little cooked grain, such as rice or buckwheat, and fruits. Eliminate all fats, sugars, alcohol, and refined foods. During the fast, drink six to eight glasses of still, bottled water daily. When you have completed the seven days, return to your regular diet gradually, avoiding fats and refined foods.

**On rising:** 1 glass hot water with a lemon squeezed into it (crush the whole lemon in a little hot water including pips, peel and seeds, and soak overnight).

**Breakfast:** Grapefruit, grapes, or other unsweetened fruit.

**Mid-morning:** Fresh fruit or vegetable juice.

**Lunch:** Vegetable broth. (Make the broth using carrots, potatoes, turnips, celery, spinach, onions, garlic and parsley and other fresh herbs, plus other vegetables in season. Cover ingredients with water, bring to a boil, simmer one hour, strain. Add a little miso (fermented soybean paste) for flavor.

**Mid-afternoon:** Fruit juice diluted with still, bottled water; or a piece of fruit.

**Dinner:** Three steamed vegetables.

**After dinner:** Herbal tea (such as chamomile or alfalfa with a little honey) or dandelion coffee.

## YOGA

Gentle exercise is probably one of the kindest things you can do with your body and spirit, and probably the best known form of gentle exercise is yoga — a non-invasive practice that is easy to do whenever it suits you.

Yoga originated in India about 5,000 years ago. It is now widely practiced all over the world as a philosophy of life. The word yoga comes from the Sansrit word *yuj* meaning "union, or to bind." This is the essence of yoga — to unify the physical body with the mind and the vital energy that flows within us all.

Yoga utilizes a number of basic techniques that combine breathing, consciousness and body awareness to bring about health, tranquillity and a sense of harmony.

Medically and scientifically proven in various research programs, yoga has been used successfully for all sorts of conditions from physical ailments to stress disorders.

Yoga encourages self-healing, strength of body and clarity of mind. This inevitably boosts the healing process, while complementing other health therapies.

Yoga is a form of meditation and meditation helps clarify the meaning of our life and our personal reality. It helps provide inner harmony and peace of mind and enables us to be more aware and "centered." Throughout history, people have strived to find health, harmony, and happiness in life. As the ancients have shown us, one way we can achieve this is by calming the mind. A calm mind helps in achieving harmony within the body.

## PRACTICAL HOME REMEDIES

### Aches and Pains

Age-old treatments include regular warm baths with a few drops of lavender, rosemary or wintergreen oil, or a handful of chamomile leaves added; and warmed cabbage leaves applied to particularly sore spots and then covered with a woolen cloth.

Garlic sliced and worn inside the socks is said to bring relief for all aches and pains.

### Acne

Many folk practitioners advocated fasting and the avoidance of water on the skin. The yolks of hard boiled eggs were pierced with wire and held over a candle. As small drops of yolk oil appeared they were collected and applied as an ointment at night, until the condition cleared.

### Bad Breath

Wormwood tea is an excellent remedy for a furred tongue and bad breath. Or try taking charcoal tablets. The ancients regularly used bits of charcoal from the fire, pounded and mixed to a paste with a little honey and water, to alleviate the after effects of too much rich food.

### Bleeding Gums

To prevent or treat bleeding gums and to remove yellow stains, grind some fresh sage leaves together in a mortar with sea salt. Dry the mixture in a slow oven until it is hard and then pound it to a powder. Rub or brush this over the teeth both morning and evening.

## Bronchitis

"A poultice of marshmallow and peppermint leaves, with a little warmed tallow from candles or some warmed oil, should be applied in a linen cloth to the chest, in the morning and evening, and gives relief. Drink tea made from thyme and coltsfoot, and rest well."
OLD ENGLISH REMEDY, C. 1750

## Bruises

"Rub gently with a piece of rag or wool dipped in olive oil, and then cover with a compress saturated with the oil. This gives instant relief, and is better than arnica."
MRS THEO P. WINNING, *The Household Manual*, C. 1899

## Burns

Break an egg, mix the white and yolk, smear over the burn and apply any sort of strong alcohol. A skin will form, soothing the pain and promoting healing.

## Colds

Grate fresh horseradish, add the juice of two lemons, a crushed clove of garlic and a pinch of cayenne pepper. Add hot water, and a teaspoon of honey. Drink three times a day.

## Cuts and Wounds

There is an old belief that cuts can be healed through the application of cobweb. This may stem from the absorbent abilities of the cobweb. If there's nothing else around, try applying honey. Honey has antibiotic and antiseptic properties and assists in wound healing.

## Cystitis

Take the cornsilk from corn cobs, add some alfalfa, and make a tea. This is a safe, natural soother for that burning pain.

## Earache

Try a few drops of warm olive oil in the ear. It has worked for centuries.

## Depression

The ancient Greeks believed that the herb of courage, borage, steeped in wine, was a sure remedy for depression. This pretty, easy-to-grow garden plant can still help, as a tea or salad ingredient, for any "feeling low" conditions.

## Diarrhea

An old Siberian remedy advocated heating a brick in the oven, covering it with a towel, and sitting on it. The brick should be as hot as can be endured. Sit on it until the brick cools down. The treatment may be repeated in an hour but should not be necessary.

If this doesn't work, the Siberians advocated taking dried, powdered chicken-stomach skin with food, once or twice a day (one stomach for each dose). The skin should be dried in the sun. The only safe remedy for children, though, was the thick residue of boiled rice, strained through cheesecloth.

## Fatigue

The Chinese have been benefiting from the powers of royal jelly, the food of the queen bee, for centuries. Its unique properties increase energy and boost the immune system.

## Flatulence
Charcoal is a great leveler for this condition, as is fennel seed. You should also examine your diet, as something is out of balance.

## Freckles and Blemishes
Lemon juice, a natural bleach, is still used around the world.

Another widely used ancient remedy is to rub the skin with hot tea, twice a day, or try an infusion of cucumber seeds soaked in pure alcohol for 12 hours, applied twice daily.

## Hemorrhoids
Grated raw carrots, taken frequently and in quantity with each meal, was one way European folk medicine practitioners helped this condition.

The Chinese used suppositories cut from fresh potatoes, inserted into the anal canal and left there for the day. A Persian remedy tells of using an anal steam bath. Sit above a very hot brick to which raw garlic pieces have been added. As the garlic cooks the afflicted area is healed by the rising smoke.

## Headaches
"Put a little salt on the tongue, and washing it down with a drink of warm water. It is the best cure we have found. Some people think it will make them vomit, but it will not. It cures the headache almost as soon as you drink it."
Early twentieth century English Remedy

## Hiccups
A traditional Russian remedy is to apply a mixture of dry mustard and vinegar to the tongue, coating half of it. Unpleasant, perhaps, but effective.

## Insomnia
A glass of dill pickle juice, sweetened with honey and taken with a little warm water half an hour before bed can produce a sound sleep.

A Caucasian remedy recommends using grated horseradish, with a little dry mustard added, as compresses on the calves of the legs before bed. It is said to take the blood away from the brain, thus inducing sleep.

## Mastitis
Apply a refrigerated cabbage leaf to the breast. Hold in place with a bra or bandage. Relief will be instantaneous.

## Nausea
An old folkloric remedy tells us to try two teaspoons of anise seeds with an equal amount of clear honey in a glass of water. Boil for ten minutes, cool, strain and take several tablespoons when necessary.

## Nerve Problems
Oats are one of the finest nerve strengtheners. They are a source of protein and are particularly rich in B vitamins and minerals. A bowl of porridge for breakfast is an effective way to combat stress at the start of each day.

## Ringworm
"Get some carbonate of soda and strong vinegar, mix and put on the ringworm. A few

applications will kill the disease, and it is a remedy that is in every home."
*The Leader Spare Corner Book*, 1930

## Stings and Bites

Remove the sting and then apply garlic juice frequently. This will stop the pain and reduce the swelling.

Another old European remedy is to moisten a piece of cloth with fresh urine and apply it to the sting.

## Stitch

"For a stitch in the side, apply treacle mixed with a very hot potato."
Golden Recipes, *Knowledge is Power*, nineteenth century

## Stye

Home remedies include rubbing the stye lightly with a cleaned garlic clove; rubbing it with the moisture collected from a steamed-up window; and circling it with a wedding ring three times and having your partner kiss it afterwards.

## Sunburn

A traditional European remedy is to smear the yolk of a raw egg over the afflicted part of the skin, allowing it to dry, and then removing the "skin" with gentle soap and water after half an hour. The results are said to be amazing.

## Tired Eyes

Wash the eyes with a weak decoction of raw onion with some honey added, or try putting on a compress of cottage cheese at night.

## Toothache

"Failing oil of cloves, a very painful toothache should receive the alcohol treatment, usually whiskey (neat) applied direct. Also a good old-fashioned cure, which succeeds often when everything else fails, is to dip a small piece of strong brown paper in whiskey, sprinkle it with pepper and apply to the face where the pain is. Cover with a flannel bandage; it does not blister the skin."
*The Australian Household Manual*, 1899

## Warts

The milky sap of the dandelion flower is a well-known remedy, used throughout history. Another common gypsy remedy, still effective, is to sell someone else your wart. You must pay an agreed amount of money to someone else, specify a date at which the wart will go, and at the appointed time it will disappear.

The Russians advocate soaking a slice of raw onion in vinegar for two hours, applying it to the wart and bandaging it tightly. Within a few days it should come out, root and all.

## Worms

Fresh garlic is probably the best preventative here. A widely used European treatment was to take a quarter of a pound of cleaned pumpkin seeds in the morning on an empty stomach, mixed with blackcurrant juice, followed half an hour later by a broth of boiled garlic, then an hour later by a dose of castor oil. For the rest of the day abstain from food, rest and stay near a toilet.

# A-Z

## OF COMMON
## MODERN AILMENTS

Throughout history humans have coped with a wide range of health problems ranging from infections to functional disorders, metabolic disorders and degenerative diseases. Not so long ago our major concern was with the many deadly infections that were rife. For example, more people died in the influenza epidemic that followed the World War II than died in the war itself. Since then, with better hygiene, sanitation and diet, complemented by the development of vaccination and antibiotics, our focus has shifted.

We now know that we are what we eat, breathe and think. Or one could say that our state of health is the result of the fine balance between physical, psychological, physiological, social, environmental and spiritual factors.

Today there is certainly a greater prevalence of the degenerative diseases (such as cardiovascular disorders and arthritis), immune diseases (such as allergies), and metabolic diseases (such as diabetes). This is a cause for serious concern. These diseases seem to be developing earlier in these modern times than they did several decades ago and are thus more serious. They probably result from our current way of life. One consideration is our Western diet. It seems dietary intake is a major factor in conditions such as diabetes, gout and cardiovascular disease. Another influential factor, over which we have little control, is environmental pollution. Air pollution is a worsening problem, and our fruits, vegetables and meats are often full of chemicals, some safe and some dangerous. The body absorbs all these chemicals and presents with a range of illnesses as a consequence. In addition, the way that many of us live results in high stress levels, which in turn can seriously affect our health.

While many of our "modern ailments" are ones that have been known throughout history, there are others that are increasing in prevalence, such as chronic fatigue syndrome, allergies and arthritis. In this section of the book we have listed those ailments that we feel are most common at present.

Ancient remedies are coming into their own once more, with a growing number of people turning to balancing therapies as they view health issues more holistically. A holistic approach entails healing by way of lifestyle and through natural means of preventing and treating disease.

In this part of the book you can look up whatever ailment is troubling you and read about ways to treat it both through the use of modern medicine and through using herbs. Advice is also given on a range of other useful natural remedies. You can then turn to the HERBAL REMEDIES section of the book (pages 12–81) to learn the properties of the indicated herbs in more detail, and discover the many ways they can be used.

# ALLERGIES

Allergies are disorders of part of the immune system. Our immune system responds to an allergen as if it were a threat to us rather than something relatively harmless, and produces the chemicals (histamines) that give us a typical allergic reaction. Common allergens include dust mites, pollens, molds, dog and cat hair, insect stings, some drugs, and foods such as milk, eggs, wheat, peanuts and fish.

There are also symptoms which resemble those of an allergy that arise from such factors as stress, cold, or wearing tight clothing. In general, the onset of allergies occurs in childhood — in other words, we become sensitized at an early age.

**SYMPTOMS:** Typical allergic reactions include itchiness, a rash, hives, dizziness, wheezing and chest tightness, coughing and even loss of consciousness. Acute food allergies may produce swelling, wheezing, diarrhea and vomiting. Asthma, hayfever, rhinitis and conjunctivitis are all well-known allergic reactions, as well as atopic eczema. Occasionally, an allergic reaction may be life threatening and immediate medical attention is required.

**TREATMENT:** The first step is to try to identify the allergen and then avoid it. Most children grow out of their food allergies by the age of six or seven years — except to fish and peanuts, which can persist to adult life. Breast feeding for the first six months helps reduce wheezing and eczema in young children. The ubiquitous dust mite is difficult to avoid but certain measures can be tried. If symptoms still persist after two months of concerted allergen avoidance and medical therapy, then allergen immunotherapy or desensitization is useful, especially for grass pollens and to a lesser degree for dust mites.

Medical therapies include antihistamines which give symptomatic relief. Sodium cromoglycate is a good preventative and is usually used locally, that is, as inhalants (asthma), nasal sprays or eye drops. Occasionally it is used orally for food allergies if complete avoidance is impossible.

**HERBAL TREATMENT: Garlic**, a natural blood purifier; **echinacea**, to strengthen the immune system; **elder flower**, for its anticatarrhal and anti-inflammatory powers; **witch hazel** for its astringent, tonic and slightly sedative qualities and **psyllium** for soothing any inflammation. Many other herbs may also assist, depending on the symptoms.

**OTHER USEFUL NATURAL REMEDIES:** Helpful supplements include vitamin E, which has antihistamine properties, and vitamin C with bioflavonoids, which lowers elevated histamine levels. Different allergies are treated in different ways. Successful treatments include the elimination of certain foods, acupuncture, the use of homoeopathic or herbal medicines, relaxation techniques, meditation and visualization. It is best to see your practitioner for an individual assessment.

# APPETITE LOSS

Lack of appetite or an inability to eat have both social and medical causes. Socially, they may be due to the taste of food, the way it has been prepared, or to the person not having had enough to eat in early childhood. Or there may be underlying physical or psychological causes. Appetite loss may be short term and associated with infection, trauma or surgery. Potentially more serious conditions include malabsorption (seen particularly in small bowel disorders), ulcers and difficulty in swallowing. Anorexia nervosa in adolescents, fadism, depression, grief and dementia are also important factors to consider. Any chronic illness or metabolic disorder may cause this condition. Drugs (medicinal or illegal), smoking, alcohol and other poisons can also be contributing factors.

**SYMPTOMS:** A multitude of disorders result in loss of appetite or anorexia, so the main task is to ascertain the underlying cause. If a person loses more than five percent in weight without dieting it should be taken seriously, and if they lose more than ten percent they should be considered malnourished. In children, a failure to gain weight should be taken seriously and investigated.

**TREATMENT:** This is determined by the underlying disorder. If appetite loss continues over a period of time, professional help should be sought. In general, it is believed that anorexia nervosa has psychological, rather than physical, origins, and that it relates to low self-esteem, distorted body image, difficulties in family relationships, or peer group pressure to conform to the fashionable stereotype that thin is better. Ninety percent of reported cases occur in adolescent girls or women. Counseling or psychotherapy may be the most effective form of treatment, although dietary factors and some naturopathic remedies may assist.

In cancer and other debilitating diseases, loss of appetite is one of the most troublesome symptoms. The appetite can usually be restored by treating pain, nausea and psychological factors, depending on the primary indications.

**HERBAL TREATMENT:** Many herbs assist in encouraging the appetite, including **yarrow, devil's claw, dandelion, gentian, chamomile, ginseng, alfalfa, licorice, milk thistle, peppermint, psyllium, feverfew, slippery elm** and **rosemary**.

**OTHER USEFUL NATURAL REMEDIES:** Dr. Bach's Flower Remedies, used for treating states of mind and underlying emotional conditions, may be particularly beneficial for treating this condition. Vitamin C, B-complex vitamins and some amino acids may help, as well as zinc supplements, homeopathy, acupuncture, traditional Chinese medicine and relaxation therapies.

# ARTHRITIS

Arthritis is the modern term for a condition which has been known to humankind for thousands of years; in ancient times it was frequently known as rheumatism, the name having derived from *rheo* (to flow), as it was believed the disease progressed from a disorder in the "humors" of the body, following the wrong track of the body's muscles, causing the excruciating pain in joints. In Culpepper's time, in the early seventeenth century, it was believed that one of the primary causes was "the taking of colds, or obstructing perspiration."

A wide spectrum of joint diseases are known as arthritis. Osteoarthritis is a degenerative disorder in which the cartilage in the joint progressively thins and breaks up, leading to complete loss of function in the joint. Anything that damages the joint surfaces can result in a predisposition to osteoarthritis, including trauma, misalignment and fractures. Osteoarthritis affects the knees (most commonly), hands (especially the thumb), hips and spine. Rheumatoid arthritis is an autoimmune disease with an hereditary association (the ratio of females to males is 3:1) which damages the synovial membrane of the joint and later the cartilage. It may involve any large joint, including the upper spine, wrists, hands and knees and can lead to marked joint deformity.

**SYMPTOMS:** Pain is the earliest symptom and occurs especially at rest and after overuse. Osteoarthritis is a very common disease of the elderly. Joints become stiff in the mornings and after resting; sometimes the condition is worse at night or in cold, damp conditions. Joints swell both with fluid and bony enlargements and there can be an audible grating in the joint. In rheumatoid arthritis there is often joint pain and morning stiffness which lasts more than half an hour, combined with general ill health, fatigue and fever.

**TREATMENT:** The exact type of arthritis needs to be diagnosed so that the most appropriate form of treatment can be prescribed. It is helpful to lose weight, avoid overuse, protect the joint with splinting or firm bandaging, use a cane or a walker, and wear a corset for low back disease or a collar for neck disease. Regular exercise to maintain muscle power and tone is important, and modifying the home and office will help. Non-steroidal anti-inflammatory drugs (NSAIDS) may be needed, however these often affect the stomach and intestines, and analgesics may be required. In rheumatoid arthritis certain drugs may be used to induce a remission. Surgery (joint

*Crush a whole lemon, peel, pulp and seeds, and mix with water and honey. Drink on an empty stomach.*
SEVENTEENTH-CENTURY HOME REMEDY FOR ARTHRITIS

*Culpepper suggested the most effective remedy for this condition to be:*
*"Hot bricks, the vapor bath, and a decoction of 1 oz. of horseradish, 1 oz. of dandelion root, 2 drachms of capsicum, 2 drachms of hops, and 1 oz of yarrow, boiled in 1 quart of water. Strain, and take a wineglassful six times a day."*

replacement) may be necessary, and sometimes tendon repairs or the excision of badly damaged bone are needed.

**HERBAL TREATMENT:** The most effective form of treatment will depend on the diagnosis, but any of these herbs may prove useful. **Aloe vera** for its soothing qualities; **celery seed** for its ability to eliminate uric acid; **thyme** for its ability to soothe nerve pain and to stimulate circulation; **willow bark** for its ability to soothe pain and inflammatory conditions; **gentian** for many arthritic conditions; **alfalfa** for its ability to eliminate uric acid; **devil's claw**, arguably the most powerful antiarthritic and analgesic of them all; **St. John's wort** for many forms of nerve pain; **ginger** as a soothing compress or ointment; **chamomile** for its calming and soothing qualities; **elder flower** for its anti-inflammatory and antirheumatic effects; **rosemary** oil externally for rheumatism or any muscular or joint pain.

**OTHER USEFUL NATURAL REMEDIES:** With regards to diet, particularly avoid the deadly nightshade family which includes potatoes, tomatoes, peppers, eggplant (aubergine) and tobacco, and avoid citrus fruits other than lemons. Massaging with comfrey or rue ointment, or the application of warmed cabbage leaves to the afflicted area and then covered, may bring relief. Another ancient remedy still widely used is stinging nettle tea to which Swedish bitters have been added. Swedish bitters or castor oil added to a warm compress and left on the afflicted area for four hours a day provides great benefit. Hot socks filled with salts and alternating hot and cold compresses on a painful joint are also helpful.

Miso, a fermented soybean product, has long been used in Japan in the treatment of arthritis and as a general alkalizing tonic for the circulation.

*"Take a quart of milk, boil it and turn it with three pints of small-beer; then strain the posset on seven or nine globules of stallion's dung tied up in a cloth, and boil it a quarter of an hour in the posset — drink; when it is taken off the fire press the cloth hard, and drink half a pint of this morning and night hot in bed; if you please you may add white wine to it".*
THE COMPLEAT HOUSEWIFE, 1753

# BALDNESS
## (ALOPECIA)

Alopecia means hair loss, in any amount, from any hairy body part. Baldness may be a prolonged change or permanent in those with a genetic predisposition. Hair follicles grow faster than any other part of the body and are easily affected by emotional stress and physical disease, although there is often a delay factor. For instance, a woman may lose hair for one to six months following childbirth, or a person may lose hair four weeks to three months after having a fever. Hair loss is also caused by thyroid disease, dieting, gout, arthritis, fungal infections, dandruff, the oral contraceptive pill, menopause and other pharmaceutical drugs, low serum iron, dietary deficiencies and high doses of vitamin A. Alopecia areata is the loss of large chunks of hair, sometimes resulting in total loss.

SYMPTOMS: The male pattern of baldness — loss of hair from the front or temple hairline, is the most common. For females, there is generally central loss, while the frontal hairline is maintained. More than 50 hairs on a brush or in the shower drain suggests a problem and can cause feelings of social anxiety and loss of self-esteem.

TREATMENT: Hair reflects our inner health — it can become dry, brittle or greasy as a result of what we eat and drink, from stress, or from a variety of environmental factors. It is important to eliminate any underlying diseases or medications as the cause of hair loss.

Medications to block male hormones have been tried as a treatment but have many side effects, especially for men. Hair transplantation is another option that suits some.

Simple measures include checking whether any chemicals applied to the hair (or taken internally) are causing the problem, avoiding excessive shampooing, avoiding pulling the hair too tightly, and not brushing too often. Don't brush your hair for more than 100 strokes, whatever Grandma may have told you.

HERBAL TREATMENT: **Rosemary**, regularly massaged in for its tonic and circulatory benefits on the scalp and hair follicles; **yarrow**, for its powerful action on the circulatory system; **thyme**, as a strengthening tonic for the scalp to help prevent hair loss; **aloe vera** as a gel or shampoo; **tea tree** as an oil or shampoo.

OTHER USEFUL NATURAL REMEDIES: Hair is made of protein (as are the nails), so eat lots of protein. Rinse the hair and massage the scalp regularly with an infusion of stinging nettle. Supplements of vitamin A, zinc, B-complex and vitamin C may be beneficial. A decoction of walnut tree leaves, massaged frequently into the scalp, is also of great assistance for hair loss.

# BRUISES

Bleeding into the tissue may result from vessel wall fragility, low blood platelet levels or deficiency in our blood clotting factors. Vascular or platelet disorders are characterized by spontaneous bleeding (including small, purplish spots) and easy bruising into the skin and mucous membranes. Coagulation disorders are usually associated with bleeding into the joints and muscles. Severe inherited disorders are picked up in infancy, but if they are mild they may show later with excess bleeding after trauma, surgery, tooth extraction and so on.

**SYMPTOMS:** A bruise caused by a blow shows characteristic discoloration, swelling and pain. Ecchymoses are bluish discolorations in the skin and mucous membranes caused by fragile vessels. They often occur in the elderly, especially on the backs of the hands, with no apparent cause. Petechiae are pinhead purple or red spots caused by tiny hemorrhages. They do not blanch with pressure.

**TREATMENT:** Treatment depends upon accurate diagnosis. Although many people say they bruise easily, only a few have an underlying blood disorder. If bruising is out of proportion to the degree of trauma, then suspect a clotting disorder. If bruising is unexplained then other causes should be considered, such as infection; an allergic response; liver or kidney failure; bone marrow disease; drug use (such as steroids, anticoagulants and aspirin); malnutrition (especially scurvy) in persons living alone or on an "ulcer" diet; and abuse — either self-inflicted or caused by others.

Immediate application of cold will help reduce spread and swelling in an injury. No drug prevents bruising but if aspirin or aspirin-containing drugs were being taken they should be stopped. Creams which break down clotting should be applied immediately and then two to three times daily help to reduce the amount of bruising visible.

**HERBAL TREATMENT: Witch hazel**, used externally, for its astringent and healing abilities; **aloe vera**, for its immediate soothing effect; **elder flower**, as an ointment from the leaves and flowers; **calendula** which helps any wound; **yarrow**, for its beneficial effects on the circulation; **horse chestnut**, to speed the healing; **rosemary** oil, for its tonic benefits.

**OTHER USEFUL NATURAL REMEDIES:** Arnica is another particularly useful cream or ointment for bruises, and may also be taken homoeopathically to assist in rapid healing and reduction of pain. Comfrey ointment may also shorten the healing time. Increasing vitamin K intake is particularly beneficial for those who bruise easily — this can be done by eating 6 oz. (150 g) of yogurt daily. Vitamin C with bioflavonoids, either in foods or as supplements, will support the blood vessels, and supplements of zinc and vitamin A may also assist healing.

# BURNS

Burns are an injury to the tissues with the breakdown of tissue proteins, fluid edema and loss of fluid from the cells and blood vessels. They can be caused by heat, radiation, chemicals or electricity. The depth of a burn depends on the intensity and duration of the cause. In superficial burns, regeneration occurs rapidly from uninjured skin elements. Deep burns, with destruction of deeper layers, repair slowly from the wound edge and can contract into disfiguring and disabling scars.

**SYMPTOMS:** In first-degree burns the skin is red and swollen, and the area is sensitive to touch and moist. There are no blisters and healing time is about one week. Second-degree burns show blisters and the skin has sensation. Recovery takes two to three weeks. In third-degree burns the skin is completely destroyed and looks white or black and leathery. Hairs can be pulled out easily and a pinprick cannot be felt. This requires immediate hospitalization.

**TREATMENT:** Immediate care should include removing any clothing associated with the burn and applying cold water or ice for up to 45 minutes to prevent further extension of the burn and reduce the associated pain and swelling.

Wounds should be cleaned with diluted iodine solution. If possible, elevating the affected areas above heart level will reduce swelling. Analgesics may be required. Topical antibacterial agents should be applied with a sterile applicator. Wounds should be dressed and changed daily, with complete removal of the previous day's topical medication. If the burn involves a joint or is second degree, then splinting may be required. Skin grafting is often necessary in third-degree burns, together with compression bandaging.

**HERBAL TREATMENT: Aloe vera,** probably nature's most famous burn soother; **elder flower** ointment, which helps burns and sunburn, **tea tree** as a soothing cream or diluted oil; **willow bark**, as a wash externally or a pain-killer internally; **witch hazel**, for its astringent and tonic properties; **calendula**, for its antiseptic properties; **St. John's wort**, for all wounds; **garlic** and **echinacea**, taken internally to help prevent infection; **marshmallow**, particularly known for soothing irritated tissue; **raspberry leaf**, used externally as a gentle wash; **rosehip tea**, for its high vitamin C content.

**OTHER USEFUL NATURAL REMEDIES:** In a first-aid situation, bathing the wound in a strong solution of tannins (the gum or galls from oak, or the bark of any deciduous tree, or very strong household tea), and then reapplying frequently will provide the formation of a temporary "skin" over the burn. High doses of vitamin C with bioflavonoids, and supplements of zinc, vitamins A and E will also promote rapid healing. Externally, a combination cream of St. John's wort, calendula and comfrey, or vitamin E cream, will help provide scar-free healing.

# CATARRH
## (INCLUDING SINUSITIS)

Catarrh is an excessive discharge of mucus from the upper respiratory tract and can be caused by many conditions. The mucus may be copious and watery, as when you have a cold, or thick and scanty with more inflamted mucous membranes. Catarrh can also be related to infections, allergies and an inappropriate diet. Sinusitis, which is often difficult to differentiate from a cold, involves acute or chronic inflammation caused by viruses, bacteria or fungi; by allergies or trauma; by a dental root abscess; or a foreign body in the nose. It may also represent disturbances of the processes of assimilation and elimination, as well as of the respiratory system.

SYMPTOMS: In sinusitis the symptoms usually worsen three to four days after an upper respiratory tract infection: the nose blocks and there is a discharge of thickened, colored mucus. Smell is often lost, and there may be a headache, tenderness over the sinuses, toothache and pain behind and between the eyes. If not treated correctly, sinusitis may become chronic.

TREATMENT: Try to avoid exposure to irritants such as smoke, known allergens and pollutants, and reduce alcohol intake. Avoid dairy products as they are mucus producing. Oils used as inhalants or chest rubs, such as eucalyptus and tea tree, are helpful. Steam inhalation reduces swelling and helps decongestion. Infection may need to be controlled by antibiotics. Short-term sprays that reduce swelling also help, as do analgesics.

It is best to avoid swimming and flying and to treat any dental problems. As a last resort, a specialist can puncture the sinus outlets and wash out the sinuses.

HERBAL TREATMENT: **Thyme**, with its power-packed antiseptic action; **elder flower**, useful for all mucous membrane problems; **tea tree**, for its immunostimulant qualities; **witch hazel**, for its drying, astringent, tonic abilities; **garlic**, the great cleanser and decongestant; **horse chestnut**, as an expectorant; **ginger**, which stimulates the circulation and promotes perspiration; **licorice**, for soothing the mucous membrane; **peppermint**, for its stimulating and cleansing effects; **marshmallow**, to soothe irritated tissue; **rosehip**, for its high vitamin C content; **echinacea**, to help boost the immune system; **chamomile**, for its soothing and relaxing qualities.

OTHER USEFUL NATURAL REMEDIES: Helpful herbs are ground ivy, eyebright, ribwort, golden rod, coltsfoot and hyssop. Horseradish, eaten raw, will help clear the sinuses. Fenugreek tea is an excellent cleanser and promotes elimination. Supplements of B-complex vitamins, high doses of vitamin C with bioflavonoids, zinc, iron, and vitamin A, which strengthens the mucous membranes, are all helpful.

# CHRONIC FATIGUE SYNDROME

This syndrome of symptoms, dominated by long-term fatigue, has been given many titles, including myalgic encephalomyelitis, post-viral syndrome, Royal Free disease and Lake Tahoe disease, and there has been much controversy about its existence. Its cause is obscure but several theories have been presented. It may be caused by a virus, or result from a disorder of the immune system or its regulation. It has also been suggested that it has a psychological basis, as many patients have co-existing depression.

The predominant symptom of this condition is extreme exhaustion, but there may be many other asssociated and seemingly unrelated symptoms. Interestingly, the most frequently affected people are often active, busy and seemingly well-adjusted people in their late twenties or early thirties; hence it's unjustified twentieth-century definition of "yuppie flu." This condition may have been around since the beginning of time — and yet, we still don't know enough about it to classify it or cure it.

Perhaps the frequent "indispositions" of women in the Middle Ages, or the aches and pains of peoples all over the world all through history, could have been symptoms of this mysterious condition, which is only now being recognized and evaluated scientifically.

Hippocrates was probably one of the first recorded physicians to try to change the wide-spread medical beliefs that illnesses were not not punishments for real or imaginary sins, or caused by evil spirits, but were due to natural causes. Previously, weakness or conditions such as chronic fatigue could lead to wives being discarded, sons being disowned and ordinary people being vilified as malingerers or criminals.

Hippocrates, and his fellow Greek Aristotle (born about thirty years later) began to show the world that it was the individual who should be examined, with an emphasis on case history and accuracy of observation. Medicine had begun to change direction, and although it has taken several centuries, it seems that we are at last starting to accept that conditions such as chronic fatigue syndrome may need to be evaluated from many perspectives, including environmental, genetic, dietary, psychological, and stress factors.

*"A hare's brain, steeped in wine, and given to drink — wonderfully it amends."*

GYPSY REMEDY FOR TIREDNESS, 15TH CENTURY

**SYMPTOMS:** There are a constellation of symptoms, the most important of which is debilitating muscle fatigue that lasts for at least six months and more than halves the patient's ability to undertake activities. Other features include a sore throat, a mild fever, painful and enlarged cervical and axillary glands, muscle pain, multi-joint pain without swelling, generalized headaches, depression, inability to concentrate, sleep disturbance and unrefreshing sleep.

**TREATMENT:** While it is unwise to label a condition as CFS without investigating other illnesses that have similar symptoms, its existence must be acknowledged in those people who fit the picture. One of the most difficult aspects of the illness is being recognized as a sufferer, as there is no "labeled" physical evidence and it can last for years. Treatment is by symptoms. Analgesics may be useful, and antidepressants may ease the commonly coexisting depression.

Numerous treatments have been tried for CFS, including immunotherapy by injections, long-term antibiotics, intravenous vitamin C and B12 injections, and ozone therapy. The wide range of treatments points to the fact that little is known about it.

*Parsley has long been held as an herb to help stem fatigue and debility.*
*A medieval recipe recommended that a bunch of parsley be steeped in white wine and hot water, and sipped through the day.*

**HERBAL TREATMENT:** Due to the non-specific nature of CFS, each case must be examined before effective assistance can be provided. **Echinacea**, the major immune-system booster; **garlic**, with its antiseptic and antiviral abilities; **ginseng**, which can increase the energy in extended periods of stress and fatigue; and more recently, **St. Johns wort**, for its strong antiviral effect on immuno-deficiency (particularly when combined with depression).

**OTHER USEFUL NATURAL REMEDIES:** Rest, a nourishing diet, gentle exercise and the avoidance of physical and mental stress all help. Counseling is also beneficial, assisting the person to come to terms with the chronic nature of the symptoms, and homeopathy, acupuncture, reflexology and Dr. Bach's Flower Remedies may provide relief. A variety of supplements may assist, those most frequently advocated being evening primrose oil, zinc, magnesium, vitamins A, B, C and E and some amino acids.

People suffering from chronic fatigue syndrome have often been diagnosed with poor immune system function, and can benefit greatly from using herbs and natural supplements to strengthen their immune responses. The yeast *candida albicans* is often found in greater than normal quantities in the intestines of patients with this condition, and a radical change in diet can dramatically assist some people – once again, you should consult your health practitioner (just as Hippocrates would have advised all those centuries ago) to obtain an individual prescription.

# CIRCULATION PROBLEMS

Circulatory problems are varied, ranging from minor ailments such as chilblains to major troubles that affect the heart and brain. This entry is limited to poor circulation in the limbs. This is most commonly caused by formation of atheromas or plaques within the blood vessels, and is usually associated with high blood fats (cholesterol and triglycerides), high blood pressure, cigarette smoking, diabetes, obesity, a family history of the disease, and being either a male or a post-menopausal woman. Chilblains result from excessive exposure to cold with an underlying poor circulation.

**SYMPTOMS:** Poor peripheral circulation may present with muscle pain on walking. After walking a specific distance, pain will stop you. Such pain is worse in cold weather and when you smoke. In severe cases the legs can be blue with shiny skin, loss of hair and thickened toenails. Ulcers and even gangrene may develop later. Chilblains appear as red, swollen areas which itch, burn, blister and ulcerate.

**TREATMENT:** You should walk to the point of pain, and then again as soon as possible, for a minimum of one hour per day. Cigarette smoking must be stopped. Drugs to open the small blood vessels and to thin the blood are also sometimes prescribed.

All measures that lower blood fats (lipids) help, including changes in diet, avoiding oxidized oils (such as fried foods), taking regular exercise and reducing alcohol. If these measures are insufficient, it may be necessary to use lipid-lowering drugs. If the blockage is severe, then surgery with bypass grafts is effective.

**HERBAL TREATMENT:** The most commonly prescribed herbs for poor peripheral circulation are: **Ginger**, which is warming, stimulating and antispasmodic; **ginkgo**, specifically indicated for promoting circulation of the blood; **yarrow**, for its powerful tonic and stimulant properties; **alfalfa**, another tonic herb which assists the normal clotting of blood; **dandelion**, widely used as a blood-cleanser for "sluggish" systems; **garlic,** for its ability to lower cholesterol; **celery seed**, an active body cleanser; **elder flower**, particularly for chilblains; and **thyme**, applied externally to promote blood supply.

**OTHER USEFUL NATURAL REMEDIES:** Prickly ash, stinging nettle, cayenne and chili all help to stimulate the circulation, so may be helpful. Repeatedly immersing the feet or hands into warm water, then cold water for 10–15 minutes may assist. Helpful supplements include vitamins A, C, E, B3 (niacin) and zinc. Most important, however, look carefully at your diet. Avoid all fatty and highly processed foods and eat plenty of fresh fruits, vegetables, grains, flaxseed (linseed), white meats and oily fish. Massage is of great benefit, as are reflexology treatments, acupuncture and aromatherapy.

# COLD SORES

These are the recurrent single or multiple blisters found around the mouth in Herpes I and around the genitalia in Herpes II, caused by the herpes simplex virus. After the initial infection the virus takes up residence in a nerve and lies dormant until reactivated. Flare-ups occur for a variety of reasons, such as a lowering of resistance, emotional stress, exposure to wind and sun, fever, menstruation and eating certain foods such as chocolate and nuts which contain the amino acid arginine.

**SYMPTOMS:** The initial infection usually occurs in childhood when it is subclinical or very mild. Secondary infection develops usually on the lip margin, mucous membranes or next to the nostrils. Their emergence is often preceded by a pricking sensation and associated swelling, then the blisters grow, rupture, crust and heal. The whole process usually takes seven to ten days.

The initial infection of genital herpes is more severe and recurrence is more common. This infection usually only occurs in sexually active people.

**TREATMENT:** First confirm the diagnosis, as other infections can give a blistery look around the mouth. Drying agents, such as surgical spirit will help to crust the lesions and reduce discomfort, and ice reduces the swelling. Povidone iodine paint has antiviral action and a drying effect, and should be applied frequently.

The aim of treatment is to enhance the body's resistance, so take high doses of vitamin C with bioflavonoids in the prodrome (the first onset of symptoms).

Specific anti-herpes creams can be applied in the prodome and for the first few days, or early treatment with tablets in Type I, or double dose for Type II, can be helpful. This works best on Type II, but has a role in both Types I and II in immunocompromised patients.

**HERBAL TREATMENT: Tea tree** oil, **St. Johns wort** and **aloe vera**, applied externally; **garlic**, **echinacea**, **ginseng**, **rosemary**, **chamomile** and **thyme** to assist internally.

**OTHER USEFUL NATURAL REMEDIES:** High doses of vitamin C, B-complex, zinc and the amino acid lysine have been shown to be very beneficial. The virus usually takes hold when the immune system is depressed, or when there are higher than normal stress levels, so try to eat a healthy, balanced diet and get plenty of rest and exercise. Always use an adequate sunscreen with PABA during exposure.

*The herpes virus family is widely distributed in humans and has many presentations:*

| | |
|---|---|
| *Herpes I* | *Common cold sore* |
| *Herpes II* | *Genital herpes* |
| *Herpes III* | *Chicken pox and shingles (herpes zoster)* |
| *Herpes IV* | *Glandular fever* |
| *Herpes V* | *Cytomegalovirus* |
| *Herpes VI* | *Rose rash of infants* |

# COMMON COLD

## (INFECTIVE RHINITIS OR ACUTE CORYZA)

The term "common cold" refers to an acute, viral infection of the upper respiratory tract, that is, the nose to the upper bronchi. There are over 150 types of viruses that may cause this, which is why immunity is hard to achieve. The viruses are highly contagious, with infants and young children having the greatest number of infections. People most commonly catch colds in winter. Susceptibility increases with fatigue, emotional distress or associated allergies.

The common cold seems to be one of the banes of both ancient and modern history — it has always been around, and it seems to just keep skipping one step ahead of any form of real cure or treatment. Many remedies have been tried over many thousands of years, but the virus seems to stay one step ahead — perhaps because cold viruses are in a constant state of change, and therefore having been exposed to one variety does not necessarily make you immune to the next one that comes along. If you are run down, or your general immunity is low, you are particularly susceptible to "catching colds." If you are healthy, and all your body systems are functioning well, you won't have to bother with the "germ theory" — your immune system will protect you against the invaders.

In ancient times, it was widely believed that being physically cold or getting wet or damp would cause a cold; today, it is thought that stress, lowered resistance, chronic illness or debility, all of which lower the immune-system response, are the the major contributory factors to a person's coming down with a cold. Many practitioners, both ancient and modern, believe that a cold is the way the body tries to eliminate toxins, and therefore have advocated just resting and allowing your system to cleanse itself naturally.

*According to Pliny the Younger (about 100 A.D.) one of the most effective treatments for colds was "kissing the hairy muzzle of a mouse." We are unaware of clinical studies that have examined the efficacy of the treatment, but you may wish to try it out.*

**SYMPTOMS:** We all know these symptoms! The incubation time is one to three days, then there is the onset of nasal obstruction, discharge, sneezing, dry sore throat and mild constitutional symptoms (general feeling of ill health, fatigue, headaches). There is seldom fever. The cold may progress to sinusitis, otitis media (middle ear infection), or bronchitis as a secondary infection.

**TREATMENT:** There is no specific treatment, and no vaccines have yet been discovered. Analgesics may be used, and antihistamines; decongestants and nasal sprays can ease the symptoms. Antibiotics are unnecessary unless there is a secondary infection.

**HERBAL TREATMENT:** The main weapons in your "fighting a cold" arsenal are **echinacea**, the principal immune system protector; **ginger**, for its warming and cleansing properties; **yarrow**, as a tonic and to promote perspiration; **tea tree**, also an immunostimulant; **thyme**, for its antiseptic action; **witch hazel**, for its astringent action; **elder flower**, for its anticatarrhal and astringent qualities and to promote perspiration; **slippery elm** and **marshmallow**, for their soothing properties; **peppermint**, as a tea or an inhalant; **garlic**, a natural antibiotic; and **rosehip**, for a vitamin C boost.

**OTHER USEFUL NATURAL REMEDIES:** Steam inhalations are useful, as are high doses of vitamin C taken on the first day, to reduce the time of disability — one gram per hour until bowel tolerance (which is loose stools or bloating). Continue the next day with a dose slightly less than bowel tolerance. Don't forget to eat lots of garlic. Sage tea makes an effective gargle. Vitamin A or cod liver oil and a mineral supplement will also assist, as will hot lemon and honey drinks. (If you're really in a hurry to get well, add some garlic, a pinch of cayenne pepper and a few fenugreek seeds to your hot lemon and honey.)

When you have a cold, eat a light diet (particularly fresh fruit and vegetables), rest as much as possible and drink plenty of fluids (particularly water and fruit juice). A traditional and pleasant tasting herbal tea for colds and influenza consists of equal parts of peppermint, elder flowers and yarrow.

Many folkloric beliefs suggest you may be able to stave off the severity of a cold by trying the following regime at the first signs: Stay in bed as much as possible; bathe the feet in very hot water twice daily, wear clean wool socks every day and wear them to bed; abstain from all food for the first 24 hours; take three quartered grapefruits, boil in two quarts of water for 20 minutes, and drink hot (add honey if desired) as frequently as possible during the day; mix dry mustard with warm water to a paste, apply to the soles of the feet at night, bandage with flannel, and apply wool socks — leave on for an hour, remove, bathe feet in hot water, put on fresh woolen socks and walk briskly in a warm room for ten minutes.

*A cold usually lasts about a week. It has been said that, as a rule of thumb, untreated colds last a week, while medical attention can end them after seven days. If you use echinacea and other herbs you may be able to reduce the duration of a cold to four or five days.*

# CONSTIPATION

Everybody's bowel habits are different (see DIARRHEA on page 118). What is important is when there is a variation from this normal. Not only should you consider the number of stools passed, but also the effort required, the stool consistency, and the incapacity to pass stools at will. Constipation is common in the elderly. Any recent change, especially in the middle-aged or elderly, requires review by your doctor.

There are many causes, including dehydration, low fiber diet, febrile or debilitating illnesses (such as hypothyroidism and depression), pregnancy, surgery, ignoring the urge to defecate, obstructions, irritable bowel, and drugs — especially opiates, iron compounds, and aluminium-containing antacids.

**SYMPTOMS:** Constipation may be the only symptom and straining is often a feature. Abdominal discomfort occurs, often associated with bloating, and the only time wind is passed is with defecation. There may be vomiting, abdominal pain, anal pain and blood in the stools — either on the outside or mixed through the stools.

**TREATMENT:** Eat lots of fresh fruits, vegetables and bran cereals to ensure that you have plenty of fiber in your diet. A good fluid intake is essential — six to eight glasses of water a day are needed to keep you well hydrated. It helps to start the day with a glass of water and lemon juice. Increasing regular exercise and responding to the "urge" are all important. Bulking agents, such as psyllium, can help when people do not wish to change their diet, but they sometimes make constipation worse and can cause gas and bloating.

If dietary changes fail to help, gentle laxatives are the next step. These include faecal softeners such as paraffin oil or dioctyl (docusate) sodium, osmotic laxatives that pull water into the bowel, and stimulant laxatives. Suppositories and enemas help to stimulate the rectum to empty.

**HERBAL TREATMENT:** The following herbs are all helpful for this condition, so just see which works best for you: **dandelion, licorice, psyllium, slippery elm, devil's claw, thyme, ginger, senna, yarrow, aloe vera, willow bark, raspberry, marshmallow** and **chamomile**.

**OTHER USEFUL NATURAL REMEDIES:** A natural laxative, such as flaxseed (linseed), may assist with simple constipation, as will changing to a high-fiber, fresh fruit and vegetable diet, particularly if you add some bran or psyllium husks and acidophilus yogurt to your cereal every morning. Avoid coffee and foods that are high in fats or highly processed. Regular exercise is important, too.

# COUGH

A cough is a sudden forcible and audible explosion of air from the lungs. It is a protective reflex action, which may be induced voluntarily and voluntarily inhibited. Our brain has a cough reflex center which responds to any irritation of the pharynx, larynx and trachea (be it mechanical or chemical); helps clear the lungs, bronchi and trachea of irritants and secretions; and prevents breathing foreign material into the lungs. A cough is a common symptom of diseases of the lungs, ears and heart.

**SYMPTOMS:** It is often the accompanying features that are helpful in defining a condition with cough; for example sputum, blood, pain, breathlessness, wheeze, a seasonal component or constitutional symptoms (general feeling of ill health, fatigue, headaches). A cough may be dry, wet, paroxysmal or persistent. A cough that lasts for more than two months may be an indication of serious underlying illness and should be investigated.

**TREATMENT:** Specific therapy to treat the underlying cause of the cough is the most effective form of treatment. A cough that produces sputum should not be suppressed unless it exhausts the patient and prevents sleep and rest. Cough supressants suppress the brain's cough reflex center. Codeine is useful, especially if the cough is painful, and helps to dry the bronchial mucus membrane.

Demulcents (soothing agents) can form a coating over irritated throat mucous membranes, and come in the form of syrups or lozenges, such as honey and glycerine. Expectorants liquify and increase the amount of secretions, which soothe the mucous membranes and aid in coughing up mucus. Antihistamines have little use as they tend to dry the throat.

**HERBAL TREATMENT: Elder flower**, which is anticatarrhal and astringent; **feverfew**, as an expectorant; **thyme** and **echinacea**, for their antiseptic qualities; **chamomile**, as a soothing antispasmodic; **licorice**, **slippery elm** and **marshmallow** for their soothing, emollient qualities; **raspberry leaf**, to help the pain; **garlic**, for its antiseptic blood-purifying ability; **rosehip**, for its high vitamin C.

**OTHER USEFUL NATURAL REMEDIES:** Any known environmental irritants should be avoided, and adequate hydration is essential. Humidifying the air with sprays or a steam inhalation is useful. Oils such as eucalyptus, Friar's balsam, rosemary and chamomile can be added to the water for inhalation.

Coltsfoot tea with honey and lemon, taken three or four times a day, is highly beneficial.

*In Russia, fresh ox blood was often used as a remedy for coughs and asthma. But an easier and more popular remedy was the inhalation of steam from well-boiled potatoes with a few added pine needles.*

# CYSTITIS

This is an inflammation of the urinary bladder. It is common in women who, because of their short urethra, are more prone to infection. It is sometimes related to sexual activity (hence the term "honeymoon cystitis"). However, it is also quite common in children and in men, sometimes as a result of anatomical abnormalities of the urinary tract. It also occurs as urinary incontinence and in women who are pregnant, are taking the oral contraceptive pill or who have ill-fitting diaphragms. Diabetics are prone to suffer with it. The most common bacteria involved are those from the bowel, so personal hygiene and wiping front to back is important.

Cystitis is due to bacteria that can reproduce rapidly in the warm urine. The bacteria usually enters the bladder by coming up the urethra from outside the body.

*The study of urine is an ancient medical practice. It is an important component of the intricacies of traditional Chinese medicine diagnosis as well as Ayurvedic medicine. Early Indian doctors recognized diabetes mellitus by the sweetness of the urine on sipping it.*

Slackness of the muscle ring that controls the release of urine from the bladder can also allow bacteria to enter the bladder. This damage may be caused by childbirth or prolapse of the womb, and may eventually cause incontinence with a cough or laugh.

**SYMPTOMS:** Many women are familiar with that acute burning sensation on urination, frequency (often every half hour or less), urgency, night urination, and discomfort and tenderness in the bladder region. The urine may be cloudy and unpleasant smelling. Sometimes there is fever and rigors (uncontrollable shaking) especially if the infection has traveled to the kidneys. These symptoms of fever and rigors can occur in children who may not have any bladder symptoms and very few constitutional symptoms.

**TREATMENT:** First, it is best to have the urine checked for infection. An infection is likely if the urine is smelly, cloudy or blood stained.

Increase fluid intake to flush the system, and make the normally acidic urine more alkaline by eating plenty of fresh fruit (other than citrus) and vegetables and using preparations such as sodium citrotartrate. Antibiotics of the sulfur or penicillin family work best. It is recommended that the bladder be emptied before and after sexual intercourse, that cotton, rather than nylon, underwear be worn, and that soaking in a bath be avoided by women with recurrent cystitis.

*The urinal remained the symbol of the medical profession until well into the eighteenth century.*

*About five percent of women have bacteria in the bladder with no symptoms. About one-third of women will have cystitis at least once in their lives.*

Cystitis is one of the most common conditions seen by general practitioners.

**HERBAL TREATMENT: Alfalfa**, which alkalizes the urine; **slippery elm,** for its strengthening and healing qualities; **tea tree,** for its antiseptic and healing abilities; **yarrow,** for its ability to increase perspiration, astringent and tonic abilities; **celery seed** and **dandelion,** particularly indicated for cystitis; **garlic** and **echinacea,** to treat infection; **psyllium and marshmallow,** for their soothing, emollient properties; **horse chestnut** and **ginseng,** if the condition becomes chronic.

**OTHER USEFUL NATURAL REMEDIES:** Decrease irritant foods such as coffee, alcohol, citrus fruits, tomatoes, red meat, wheat and sugar, and drink lots of water and cranberry juice. Drinking extra fluid will help wash the infection out of the kidneys and bladder. The diet should be about 80 percent alkaline, so eat plenty of fruit and vegetables because almost all of them become alkaline after digestion. The herbs cornsilk and couchgrass are also particularly helpful. Useful supplements are vitamins A, E and C. A douche made from diluted cider vinegar, tea tree or acidophilus yogurt can be extremely soothing and beneficial.

*"The pain may be relieved by the application of fomentations or hot compresses to the lower porton of the abdomen and external genitals."*

THE LADIES' HANDBOOK OF HOME TREATMENT,
EULALIA S. RICHARDS

# DEPRESSION

Depression is a disorder of mood. It can be related to the events of life (reactive depression) or result from a chemical imbalance in the brain (endogenous depression), but it may also be related to stress, illness, alcohol and drugs.

Anxiety disorders may include generalized anxiety, post-traumatic stress disorder, phobias, panic disorders (most often in young females), and obsessive compulsive disorders. There may be a family predisposition, and there may be a link to personality type.

Depression, anxiety, despondency and all sorts of mood swings have affected humankind throughout recorded history. In medieval times, the earliest organized healers in England were perhaps the Druids, priestly magicians who specialized in second sight, sorcery, herbal lore and occasionally, sacrifice — sometimes all these things were needed to

*"I shall despair.*
*There is no creature loves me;*
*And if I die no soul will pity me:*
*And wherefore should they, since*
*that I myself*
*Find in myself no pity to myself?"*
RICHARD 111, SHAKESPEARE

restore balance to those affected by the melancholy which many cultures believed could take over a person's spirit. Most ancient cultures recognized it and treated it in different ways, varying from mild herbal tonics to burning at the stake; or in more recent times, electroconvulsive and deep sleep therapies. No one cause, or cure, has been established, then or now.

**SYMPTOMS:** Depression can present as a sense of worthlessness, inadequacy or guilt, difficulty in thinking and concentrating, possibly irritability and aggression. There is a loss of interest in most activities, even day-to-day tasks, disturbance of appetite and weight, tiredness, fatigue, constipation, change in menstruation, headaches, insomnia and loss of libido. Substance abuse and suicide may occur if the condition is not recognized and treated.

Anxiety disorders are an accentuation of a normal emotion: symptoms occur more frequently, more severely and are more persistent. Among the many symptoms possible are palpitations, flushing, chest pain, rapid breathing, dizziness, shaking, indigestion, nausea, diarrhea, blurred vision, sweating and a fear of dying or going crazy.

**TREATMENT:** If the depression has led to neglect of self or environment, a loss of physical health, or the risk of suicide, specialist attention may be needed or admission to hospital. Otherwise, treatment depends on the degree of depression. Mild depression is treated by counseling, psychotherapy or behavioral therapy.

Moderate depression usually requires drug therapy, starting with tricyclic antidepressants. This helps with insomnia after a few days, but the full antidepressant effect is not felt for 10 to 14 days. Other antidepressants work on a variety of chemical pathways, some of them taking up to six weeks to come to full effect.

Psychotherapy can be useful in alleviating anxiety disorders, the client either being treated individually or as part of a group. Regular exercise, relaxation and stress management techniques may be beneficial. Caffeine, alcohol and nicotine should be avoided. Anxiety relieving drugs, antidepressants and some blood pressure lowering drugs can be used to relieve symptoms such as palpitations, tremor and sweating.

**HERBAL TREATMENT:** In recent times, **St. John's wort** has been clinically proven to be as effective for mild and moderately severe depression, and some forms of anxiety, as pharmaceutical drugs. Other beneficial herbs include **valerian**, for depression, stress and anxiety; **chamomile**, the gentle relaxant; **feverfew**, particularly when associated with headaches or migraine; **celery seed**, for depression and apathy; **ginkgo**, whose main active pharmacological substance targets the brain; **ginseng**, the great pick-me-up herb; **milk thistle**, particularly with liver indications; **rosemary**, a relaxant and antidepressant.

*"If you would at all times be Merry, eat Saffron in meat or drink and you will never be sad. But Beware of eating overmuch, lest you should die of excessive Joy!"*
OLD ENGLISH REMEDY

**OTHER USEFUL NATURAL REMEDIES:** Exercise is particularly beneficial. As the circulation is stimulated, the hormone seratonin, which promotes a sense of well-being, is released to the brain. Diet should be examined carefully, as highly processed, fatty or high-sugar foods can slow down the digestion and the circulation of blood to the brain. Many therapies can help with depression and anxiety, especially homeopathy, Dr. Bach's Flower Remedies, acupuncture, relaxation, and regular massage, reflexology or aromatherapy. Effective supplements include the B-complex vitamins, vitamins C and E, zinc, magnesium and iron and evening primrose oil.

*An eastern European folk remedy suggests that once or twice weekly, patients should moisten their night clothes in salt water and go to bed in them, well covered, and stay this way until dry; then, the body was rubbed down, dry clothes applied and the patient went to bed. This was said to quickly eliminate fits of melancholy.*

# DIARRHEA

There is no clear division between normal and abnormal bowel habits. The "normal" for individuals may range from three stools per day to one stool every three days. What must be paid attention to is a change in the bowel habits for that particular person — that is, in volume, water content or frequency. Acute diarrhea is usually self-limiting and resolves within a few days. Chronic diarrhea can persist for weeks or months. Changes may hold greater significance for the elderly, for infants and the institutionalized. Look for any likely cause, such as travel to the developing world, any suspect food source, contact with anyone suffering from diarrhea, recent stress, or any possible causative medications or underlying disease.

Diarrhea has been a symptom of many conditions, for many peoples and cultures, throughout time. It may relate to many factors, but has generally always been recognized as an indication that something isn't working on the inside. There have been many folk remedies used over the centuries, but probably the most widely used remedy has been rest, fasting and plenty of fluids. It can be a symptom of many illnesses or diseases — even in ancient times, it was a major indication for plagues, dysentery, infections and fluxes, and frequently proved very hard to treat. A widespread purgative for simple diarrhea, used in many cultures, was a table-spoon of castor oil, followed by lemon juice.

One modern belief is that lactose intolerance may be a major contributing factor in chronic diarrhea, a condition which may occur in early childhood, or which may suddenly appear during the adult years. Avoiding all lactose-containing foods, especially dairy products (except yogurt), may be an easy solution in these cases.

**SYMPTOMS:** The significance of diarrhea varies according to several factors. These include fever, associated pain, stool volume (this may vary from small amounts of soft stool to large, watery stools), the nature of the feces (are they difficult to flush, do they contain blood or mucus?), the time of day when it occurs and any associated weight loss or dehydration. Infective diarrhea can vary from within one to ten hours from ingestion of suspect food, where vomiting is the main feature, to up to 70 hours later when diarrhea is the most significant feature.

**TREATMENT:** In simple diarrhea, when there is no fever and no blood, the best treatment is no treatment. This type of diarrhea usually clears up within 24 to 48 hours and it is best to allow the possible infection to be flushed out — this is the body's mechanism for removing an unwanted visitor. In more severe diarrhea, especially if it is associated with vomiting, it is important to avoid dehydration. Water, vegetable broth or diluted cordials or soft drinks can be used. Small sips which stay down are more valuable than a cup that is vomited back. Oral rehydrating solution may be given if

vomiting is not too severe. Try two pints
(1 liter) of boiled water with one teaspoon
of sugar and a pinch of salt added. It is best to
keep foods simple: fats or highly sugared foods
may worsen the diarrhea. Continue to avoid
these in the recovery phase and also avoid
caffeine, milk and antacids.

Any antidiarrheals must be used carefully as
your body may be trying to eliminate an
organism. Avoid antibiotics unless there is a
proven infection.

Diarrhea in babies or young children should
always be checked by your medical practitioner,
as should diarrhea when blood is present or
when there is fever, weight loss or dehydration.

**HERBAL TREATMENT:** A range of herbs are
useful in treating diarrhea, including **yarrow**,
**gentian**, **ginger**, **ginseng**, **horse chestnut**,
**peppermint**, **psyllium**, **raspberry leaf**,
**slippery elm**, **calendula**, **witch hazel**,
**chamomile**, **devil's claw** and **thyme**.

**OTHER USEFUL NATURAL REMEDIES:** Specific
treatments include those that increase the bulk
of the stool, such as psyllium husks (taken in
small quantities) which will absorb the water in
the stools. Pectin-rich substances, found in
ripe fruits such as apples and bananas, can also
thicken stools. Teas of meadowsweet/raspberry
leaf, or cinnamon/ginger slow down intestinal
contractions (peristalsis). Yarrow, marshmallow
and peppermint tea, which increases the tone
of your bowel muscle, will also assist recovery.
Take acidophilus yogurt two or three times a
day and avoid tea and coffee.

*Of all travelers' diarrheas,
40 to 70 percent are caused by* E. coli,
*a bacteria found in the bowel;
10 to 35 percent are of unknown
origin. Antibiotic-related diarrhea
can take up to six weeks after
treatment to appear.*

To help rest the bowel and balance the
system, go on a clear fluid diet. These fluids
can include chicken broth, consommé, miso
soup and fruit or vegetable juices. Fluids
containing natural salt and small amounts of
sugar are particularly beneficial as they help
the body replace minerals and glucose lost in
diarrhea, and help avoid dehydration. Strained
carrot juice is another excellent remedy, as it
replaces minerals and electrolytes lost during
the diarrhea. Avoid carbonated fluids, as they
may just exacerbate the gas problem. In the
recovery stage, foods such as buttermilk,
acidophilus yogurt, papaya, bananas, rice,
slippery elm powder and charcoal tablets may
all assist a speedy return to health.

*An ancient Russian remedy for
persistent diarrhea, which does not have
associated headache or fever, consists of
giving 12 large, peeled, cored and
grated apples, taken over 24 hours, one
apple every two hours, with no other
food, drink or medication.*

# ECZEMA AND DERMATITIS

The terms "eczema" and "dermatitis" both refer to inflammation of the skin surface. Such inflammations are generally caused by contact with irritants or substances in the environment, such as metals, dyes, creams, plants or rubber. Endogenous or atopic eczema (also known as the itching disease) usually occurs where there is a family history of some allergic reaction, such as asthma, hayfever or rhinitis.

These inflammations have been around for many thousands of years, although perhaps they may be more widespread today in some developed countries due to the high levels of pollutants, highly processed diets, and sedentary lifestyles — and perhaps in the developing world, due to malnourishment or disease. In medieval times in England and Europe, it was believed that the influence of the mind over the patient could lead to all sorts of bodily disturbances — thus vexation, sorrow, fear, anger, terror and so on were often believed to be predisposing conditions leading to body symptoms. Interestingly, this theory was held in many other cultures all through time; in Chinese medicine, eczema and skin rashes are closely associated with lung problems or the emotions of fear or anxiety.

**SYMPTOMS:** In the acute stage, there is redness, swelling, weeping and oozing. The chronic phase involves continued redness, crusting, scaling and thickening of the skin. The main symptom is itching, although sometimes there is just discomfort or soreness.

Infants mainly have eczema on the face, chest, scalp, neck and flexor surfaces of elbows and knees. It is blistery with much oozing, and visible scratch marks can be found.

In children aged four to ten years it appears in the folds of the neck and is more apparent on elbows, wrists and knees. Teenagers and adults tend to have dry, thickened, raised areas on the neck, inside the elbows, knees and groin, and around the eyes and forehead.

**TREATMENT:** First, it is important to obtain a positive diagnosis to ensure that it is a case of eczema and not tinea, impetigo or psoriasis. It is also necessary to treat overlying bacterial or yeast infections, if they are present, as well as the eczema. Astringents are used to cool and dry the acute weeping lesions — these include normal saline or Condy's crystals. Antihistamines may be useful to relieve the

*Native American folklore has long proclaimed the use of a teaspoon of cider vinegar and honey in hot water, taken two or three times daily, as a cure for eczema and dermatitis.*

*Folk medicine in Europe said that fresh tomato juice, not canned, regularly applied to the area is a very effective remedy in most itchings, and should be applied three times daily, then bandaged with a linen or cotton cloth.*

itching, and tar preparations may help with the itching and scaling. Corticosteroid creams or lotions for inflamed weeping areas and ointments for dry areas have a role, but should not be applied to to face, or used on infants.

**HERBAL TREATMENT: Tea tree**, the great antifungal and antibacterial healing agent; **echinacea**, a major blood-purifying herb; **aloe vera**, **marshmallow**, **raspberry** and **elder flower**, for their soothing ability; **horse chestnut**, for its anti-inflammatory properties; **witch hazel**, for its tonic and antiseptic qualities.

**OTHER USEFUL NATURAL REMEDIES:** Look for and avoid foods and environmental factors which are known triggers. Avoid hot showers and do not use soap as it is too alkaline. Keep the skin well hydrated by drinking plenty of water and using moisturizers such as cold pressed wheatgerm or apricot oil (not lanolins). Increase your intake of vitamin A, vitamin B-complex, vitamin C and zinc.

Evening primrose oil may be a useful supplement. Cool oatmeal baths will soothe the skin.

A combination of the herbs sarsaparilla, red clover and burdock made into an infusion and drunk daily may assist, as may the application of ointments of chickweed or juniper. Well pounded warmed fresh cabbage leaves, applied to the affected area twice daily and covered with a bandage, are said to relieve even the most severe symptoms. Consult a health practitioner, and try an elimination diet or cut down on all processed foods, avoid animal fats (eat oily fish and pure vegetable oils), cut out dairy products (except lacto-bacillus yogurt) and eat lots of vegetables, fruits and whole grains. Homeopathy, acupuncture, reflexology and traditional Chinese medicine may all be of benefit.

*"Boil well the dung of a gazelle in water with the rinds of pomegranates, strain off the liquor, mix well with sheep oil and apply."*

*"Take a good quantity of snails and ground salt and boyle them together and lay it on the place to relieve swelling and redness."*

OLD ENGLISH REMEDIES

# FEVER
## (HYPERPYREXIA OR HYPERTHERMIA)

Fever is an important symptom. It tells us that there is a rise in body temperature above the day-to-day functioning level and our immune system is drawing the battle lines. The cause may be infections — either the action of outside organisms or your body's defence mechanisms against them, or non-infectious — generally related to an inflammatory process or a more serious medical condition. It is important to find a possible source, such as recent exposure to infection, previous illness, injuries, recent surgery, overseas travel or drug use. Low fevers can go unnoticed, especially in young children. It may also occur on its own, known as fever (pyrexia of unknown origin. If a fever persists over a few days, or stays high over a few hours, seek medical help straight away.

**SYMPTOMS:** A fever may be the first symptom, and sometimes the only one, of an underlying problem. Get a thermometer. Use it correctly and take its reading seriously.

A high fever may have many accompanying features, including sweating, chills, rigors, uncontrollable shaking, delirium (especially in the elderly), headache, muscle pain, rash, and a rise in pulse rate and respiration. A low fever may just mean you have a cold or flu. If you're worried, see your medical practitioner immediately.

**TREATMENT:** An old theory is that the body's immune system works better with an increased temperature, so leave a low fever alone. This can be a bit risky, however, as a fever is giving us a clue that something's wrong, and fever in a child can result in febrile convulsions. Generally, though, convulsions take place because of a rapid rise in temperature and they often occur before the parent is aware that their child is really sick. Medications include those that inhibit the brain's response to fever, such as aspirin, acetaminophen, paracetamol, or non-steroidal anti-inflammatories.

**HERBAL TREATMENT:** Numerous herbs can be used to treat fever, some of which are more specific to certain types of fever than others. Herbs to try include **chamomile, elder flower, thyme, yarrow, willow bark, ginger, horse chestnut, licorice, meadowsweet, peppermint, dandelion** and **gentian**.

**OTHER USEFUL NATURAL REMEDIES:** It is best to keep cool, so do not put on extra blankets or warm clothes in summer when you think you might have a temperature. This is especially important for children. Tepid baths are worthwhile to cool the skin, and a cooling fan may help. Frequent sips of water or cool chamomile tea are also beneficial.

# FIBROMYALGIA SYNDROME

## (FIBROMYOSITIS, MYOFASCIAL PAIN SYNDROME)

This complex syndrome, which is common and often debilitating, consists of widespread musculoskeletal pain and tenderness at various sites, with associated fatigue and poor sleep. The cause is unknown. It seems to be associated with ongoing activation of pain-sensitive nerve fibers, and there is disturbed microcirculation in the muscles, so there may be an energy-deficient state as well. The information from normal movements or posture send messages to an overly sensitized system, resulting in pain and increased reflex muscle tightness.

**SYMPTOMS:** The main symptoms are widespread pain (but there may just be tender points), burning, aching, variation in severity and position, muscle ache after exercise, muscle stiffness and muscle fatigue, all of which can be dominant and interfere with daily activities. They also present at rest. The pain is present for more than three months. Associated features are sleep problems, emotional distress and general fatigue.

**TREATMENT:** Due to the complex nature of this condition it is essential to take an holistic approach. The patient must be encouraged to believe that it is not a psychological process but a sensitization of the body's pain system and that it is potentially reversible. Simple analgesics such as paracetamol, taken regularly, are the basis of management. Opiates should be avoided. Non-steroidal anti-inflammatories may be used, but are generally not very effective. Injection of local anaesthetic into the trigger points or where the muscle attaches to bone may also be useful.

**HERBAL TREATMENT:** Many herbs can assist in the treatment of this condition, depending upon the symptoms. **Elder flower**, **devil's claw**, **horse chestnut** and **gentian** are probably the most specific. Other herbs, such as **willow bark**, **valerian** and **chamomile**, may assist with pain relief.

**OTHER USEFUL NATURAL REMEDIES:** Simple lifestyle management with regular exercise and stress management may be all that is necessary. Try magnesium as well as vitamins A, E, C and B-complex. Cognitive behavioral therapy, hypnotherapy and biofeedback are all beneficial, as are acupuncture, massage, yoga and Feldenkrais technique.

# GOUT

This disease, most commonly characterized by an acute arthritis, is caused by high uric acid levels in the blood with formation of urate crystals in the joints and surrounding tissues. There is an inherited predisposition. It is usually due to the excessive production of urate, mostly from a high intake of purines in the diet — these are commonly found in alcohol, red meats and shellfish. However, gout can also occur if the kidneys have a low excretion of urate or there is kidney disease. Gout may be associated with uric acid kidney stones which can also be extremely painful.

**SYMPTOMS:** A tender, red and swollen joint — usually only one and classically the big toe with, initially, complete recovery. Occasionally there is no acute attack but only persistent low-grade joint pain. Recurrences can occur, and the arthritis may become chronic and deforming.

**TREATMENT:** This needs to be long term, especially if the underlying cause is still present. Acute attacks can be treated with non-steroidal anti-inflammatories. There is a risk that non-steroidal anti-inflammatories may create high potassium levels in the body, especially in the elderly. Colchicine is an traditional remedy and very effective, but doses close to toxic levels (causing diarrhea and vomiting) are needed in order to be effective.

Lowering urate concentration will prevent further deposition of crystals. Uric acid production may be blocked by allopurinol. The alternative is to increase uric acid excretion from the kidneys, but this must be backed up with a high urine volume, so fluid intake must be at least five pints (three liters) a day. It is best to keep the urine alkaline so sodium bicarbonate or sodium citrate should be taken. Salicylates antagonize this effect and should be avoided.

**HERBAL TREATMENT: Celery seed, alfalfa, devil's claw, elder flower, meadowsweet, milk thistle, dandelion, gentian, willow bark, ginger, peppermint** and **rosemary** are all helpful.

**OTHER USEFUL NATURAL REMEDIES:** High purine foods should be avoided, such as organ and red meats, shellfish, tomatoes, potatoes, eggplant, herrings, sardines, mackerel, anchovies, beans, salami, paté, oranges and possibly red or fortified wines. Weight loss and reduction of blood triglycerides also help.

Rest, high fluid intake and pain relief are essential, and splinting the inflamed joint may bring relief. A poultice made from stinging nettle, comfrey and rue may ease the pain. Many supplements may assist, but are best prescribed for the individual by a naturopathic practitioner.

# GUM DISEASE

Gum disease or gingivitis is chronic inflammatory disease of the supporting tissues of the teeth caused by a complex mixture of organisms. Plaque is often responsible. Other predisposing factors include malocclusion (an abnormality in the coming together of the teeth), tartar (an encrustation deposited by the saliva), impacted food, and breathing through the mouth. The rate of progression varies between individuals or within different sites in the mouth. Bleeding gums can indicate vitamin deficiency, infections or ulcers in the mouth.

**SYMPTOMS:** Gingivitis is indicated when there are red gums. There is seldom much pain but there can be bad breath and swelling which deepens the crevices between the gums and the teeth-creating pockets, and gentle probing can easily cause bleeding.

Peridontitis is a signal. There is destruction of bone and ligaments around the teeth with recession, deepening pockets, possible tooth mobility, but usually not much pain unless abscess formation occurs. This process can become chronic.

**TREATMENT:** The most important aspect is to remove dental plaque and tartar. Mouth hygiene with correct tooth brushing and cleaning between the teeth is a good habit throughout life. Toothpastes should have an abrasive effect and teeth should be brushed horizontally at the gum margin. Dental floss or toothpicks should be used horizontally. Regular professional cleaning at the dentist to remove plaque both above and below the gum line is important.

Mouth rinses may be necessary. If tooth surfaces are clean such a mouth rinse prevents about 60 percent of plaque formation. Phenolic compounds used as mouth rinses prevent up to 40 percent of plaque formation and have no long-term problems. If peridontal abscesses develop then antibiotics may be prescribed.

Persistent bleeding, discharge and pain from the gums may require surgery to gain access to the root surfaces, but if there is good plaque control and thorough dental cleaning, most cases can be resolved naturally.

**HERBAL TREATMENT: Calendula**, particularly indicated for peridontal disease; **yarrow** and **witch hazel**, for their astringent and tonic abilities; **aloe vera** and **marshmallow**, for their soothing qualities; **willow bark**, for its astringent and natural anaesthetic qualities; **tea tree**, for its antiseptic properties; **rosehip**, for its Vitamin C content; **thyme**, for its antimicrobial and anti-inflammatory abilities.

**OTHER USEFUL NATURAL REMEDIES:** Sore, bleeding gums may indicate various vitamin and mineral deficiencies, particularly vitamins A, B-complex, E, C, and some minerals. A healing gargle can be made from sage and yarrow tea, and chewing cardamom seeds may help.

A practical, effective toothpaste can be made by combining two parts of sodium bicarbonate and one part salt.

# HANGOVER

The most commonly abused drug in our society is alcohol. This is a major, potentially preventable health problem. In some cases, there may be genetic or biochemical factors in the background, but our improved and affluent lifestyles, with their associated stress factors, have created high levels of alcohol and drug taking. And, of course, the abuse of therapeutic drugs, such as tranquilizers, narcotics and amphetamines, as well as ingesting non-therapeutic drugs, such as lysergic acid diethylamide (LSD) and cannabis sativa (marijuana), can also lead to a "hangover" or altered mental state.

We all get hungover when we drink too much too quickly. Our bodies don't have a chance to break down the alcohol before our systems accumulate harmful metabolic by-products, such as the compound acetaldehyde.

*One to two glasses of red wine a day for a healthy adult male and one a day for a female reduce the risk of heart disease, although the same quantities of white wine increases cholesterol levels. Moderate wine drinkers generally enjoy greater longevity than non-drinkers or beer or spirits drinkers.*

When released into the bloodstream, acetaldehyde affects the brain and other vital organs. It is the resulting stress suffered by these organs that is your hangover.

A group of body enzymes, called ethanol dehydrogenators, take about two hours to metabolize the half fluid ounce of alcohol in a standard drink. These enzymes are active in the liver. Men, but not women, also have these enzymes in their stomachs, which help to break down 30–40 percent of alcohol. This is why men can drink more than women, even large women. Women's bodies are less tolerant of alcohol in other ways as well. They absorb alcohol more quickly when pre-menstrual and when ovulating. The contraceptive pill inhibits the breakdown of alcohol so women on the pill can get terrible hangovers.

Alcohol inhibits the body's production of the anti-diuretic hormone (ADH). Whatever quantity of alcohol you drink it will rob the body of one and a half times that amount of the body's vital water. This water takes with it valuable vitamins and minerals, causing loss of strength and energy.

SYMPTOMS: The usual hangover symptoms include headache, diarrhea, nausea, vomiting, shakiness, general body aches, depression and anxiety.

TREATMENT: The simplest solution is to avoid drinking too much. Don't over indulge on an empty stomach, and regulate the alcohol intake to one average drink per hour. Your body burns up alcohol at approximately half an

*In Germany, the traditional hangover medicine is herrings with dill and sour cream, sausages, ham — and beer.*

*Puerto Rican folk medicine extols the virtues of lemons. Not eaten, not juiced, but cut in half and rubbed under the armpits.*

ounce per hour, or one standard drink; it takes eight molecules of water to burn up one molecule of alcohol — so, your body needs a lot of water to break down the alcohol. One of the most sensible things to do is to also drink any non-alcoholic drinks — alternate alcohol with a glass of water, and you may be able to avoid that weak, headachy, fuzzy-headed feeling the next day. The morning-after symptoms may be helped by antacids (before and while drinking), or simple antidiarrheals — or try the traditional remedy of raw or soft-boiled egg. Have simple foods only the next day, such as cooked cereals, soups, rice and fresh fruit. Strong coffee, by the way, doesn't help you burn up alcohol — it only makes for a wide-awake drunk. Most of all, increase your water or fruit-juice fluid intake, and take an aspirin for the headache. And don't believe the hair-of-the-dog story, it may just get you into the mood to start again, and lead you back to where you were before.

**HERBAL TREATMENT: Milk thistle**, the number one liver protector; **feverfew**, may help with the morning-after effects of alcohol; **dandelion**, a good general liver cleanser; **rosemary**, for the sluggish morning-after feeling and for general depression from any sort of drug abuse; **psyllium**, long known as a powerful healing herb, and recently being investigated for its effects on alcohol abuse.

**OTHER USEFUL NATURAL REMEDIES:** An infusion of thyme tea, zinc tablets, high doses of vitamin C can all help with alcohol use. We need to replace vitamins, especially the B-vitamin thiamin, and also magnesium. A high protein diet may be necessary to replace amino acids; and the amino acid glutamine, given in high doses, appears to block the desire to drink alcohol.

*Shepherds on the island of Crete cure their hangovers with* kokkoretski *— sheep's intestines stuffed with chunks of lungs.*

# HEADACHE

The brain itself has hardly any pain sensors but the surrounding structures do. Headache may be due to any of the following: dilation of the blood vessels in the head, both inside and outside the skull; irritation of the brain covering, such as meningitis; irritation of the nerves; increased pressure in the skull — for example from a tumor, muscle tension (especially of neck and scalp); or psychological causes. Other more unusual causes include sinusitis, dental problems, cervical spondylosis, glaucoma (an eye disease) and other problems with eyesight, or a slow bleed from an old head injury.

Headaches can be caused by a seasonal allergy, or a sensitivity to the chemicals naturally occurring in foods. Summer colds or winter flu can bring on a headache, as can too much sun, constipation, not eating nutritiously or regularly, smoking cigarettes or drinking alcohol, tea or coffee too often. Recurring headaches, particularly the throbbing variety, are most often associated with stress and negative emotions.

The cluster headache, which afflicts more men than women, usually attacks one side of the head, and is focused on an eye socket. Cluster headaches are so called because they show up for a while and then disappear.

Sinus headaches are often felt most severely right between the eyes and less so, but still painfully, just above the inner end of each eyebrow and just below the cheekbones.

*An old English folk belief stated that "No hair, either cut or combed from the head, must be thrown carelessly away, lest some bird should find it and carry it off, in which case the person's head would ache during all the time that the bird was busy working the spoil into its nest."*

**SYMPTOMS:** Headaches only occasionally have a serious outcome, but they should never be considered trivial. If constant or occurring at regular intervals over years it is probably functional. The most severe headaches are migraines, meningitis and hemorrhages. Increasingly severe attacks may indicate the presence of a tumor. Associated features include nausea, painful sensitivity to light, fever, personality changes and nerve defects. Headaches present on waking may suggest more significant problems, especially if made worse by coughing, sneezing or straining to pass stools. In these cases seek medical advice.

**TREATMENT:** The treatment of a headache should be determined by the underlying cause. Diagnosis is often made by the history; for example, a headache from a hangover is easily recognized. Stress causes headaches, although people often do not see the connection.

*"Lavender is of a special good use for all the griefs and pains of the head and brain that proceed of a cold cause ..."*

NICHOLAS CULPEPPER, SEVENTEENTH-CENTURY PHYSICIAN AND ASTROLOGER — *THE COMPLETE HERBAL AND ENGLISH PHYSICIAN*

Tension headaches may also arise in conjunction with other causes, such as hypertension. Severe or prolonged headaches need to be reviewed by a doctor. Avoiding the causes helps, as well as reassurance that most headaches are no problem. Analgesics, such as paracetamol, together with antiemetics such as prochlorperazine often give quick relief, although analgesics seldom help with stress headaches. Antidepressants may have a role. Specific drugs, such as ergotamine, can be helpful in migraines if used at the beginning of the attack. Most headaches seem to improve more as a result of the acknowledgment and support provided rather than from the use of any specific drug.

**HERBAL TREATMENT:** Many herbs are useful in treating headaches, including **chamomile, willow bark, feverfew, ginkgo, yarrow,** **meadowsweet, rosehip** and **valerian.** Other herbs may assist if there are other underlying conditions.

**OTHER USEFUL NATURAL REMEDIES:** Massage, relaxation techniques such as regular meditation or yoga, and applying the essential oils rosemary, clary sage or lavender to the temples, or using in an oil burner or in a relaxing warm bath may help. Taking B-complex vitamins, a mineral supplement, vitamin C, and antioxidants can help with stress headaches. Eliminate highly processed and fatty foods from the diet, incorporate gentle exercise into your lifestyle, and drink plenty of water or chamomile tea.

*Feverfew was always stocked by the early monastic apothecaries of Europe and prescribed for headaches. Centuries later, one of England's great Elizabethan herbalists and healers, John Gerard, continued to sing its praises:*

*"[Feverfew is] ... very good for them that are giddie in the head, or which have the turning called Vertigo, that is, a swimming and turning in the head."*

JOHN GERARD —

*THE HERBAL*

# HICCUPS

We've all had hiccups at one time or another, and we've all been embarrassed by them, but what causes them? Hiccups are due to an involuntary spasmodic contraction of the diaphragm, together with closure of the glottis — the slit-like opening between the vocal cords. There are a multitude of causes, ranging from eating or drinking too quickly, from pregnancy, to a range of serious medical conditions including pleurisy, nerve irritation and bowel conditions.

**SYMPTOMS:** While hiccups can be common they usually last no more than a few seconds to five or ten minutes. Occasionally, they can be continuous (some may last for days) or recurrent and distressing. In such cases medical advice should be sought. Interestingly, they are more common in men.

**TREATMENT:** There are a multitude of tricks to try to stop hiccups. Increasing blood carbon dioxide inhibits them — that's why we hold our breath for as long as possible, or repeatedly breathe into a paper bag. Try swallowing crushed ice, drinking water quickly (from the back of the glass) or pushing gently on the eyeballs. Another approach is for you to stand in front of the afflicted person, hold your index finger about a foot away from the hiccuper's eyes, and say: "You must concentrate on my finger. Whatever happens, whichever way I move it, you must keep your eyes on the tip of my finger." You should keep repeating this. If the hiccuper can manage to concentrate on the finger for about a minute, you've got them. Then snap your fingers, and hey presto, no more hiccups. (This doesn't usually work with alcohol-induced hiccups.)

If hiccups are continuous and are causing distress antinausea drugs may be useful, or an antianxiety medication may assist as a muscle relaxant. For serious long-term cases, consult a doctor.

**HERBAL TREATMENT:** Herbs that have a relaxing and calming action on the nervous system may help, such as **chamomile**, **valerian**, **chamomile**, **rosemary** and **ginkgo**.

**OTHER USEFUL NATURAL REMEDIES:** Taking two teaspoons of undiluted raspberry cordial will usually take effect immediately, and a cup of dill seed tea is also often prescribed successfully.

*"Immerse the sufferer in a cold bath by the light of the moon. If there is no moonlight then a lighted candle should be placed in an adjoining room."*
MEDIEVAL CURE FOR HICCUPS

# HYPERTENSION

Hypertension is abnormally high blood pressure. Your blood pressure should not go above 150 for the systolic (top) reading or 90 for the diastolic (bottom) reading. Raised blood pressure results from either an increased resistance in the blood vessels or increased blood volume. In 90 percent of cases of hypertension there is no clear cause and these cases are called "essential." Risk factors include stress, high blood cholesterol, diabetes mellitus, a family history of hypertension, and cigarette smoking. Secondary hypertension has a specific cause. It is usually related to kidney, adrenal and thyroid disease, pregnancy or the oral contraceptive pill.

**SYMPTOMS:** There are usually no symptoms until the disease is advanced. A possible indicator of increased diastolic pressure is a headache at the back of the head in the morning, and possibly fatigue, dizziness and nose bleeds. Most symptoms are related to damage of specific organs where complications may arise.

**TREATMENT:** First, one should try non-drug methods to reduce blood pressure, especially when it is only minimally raised, for at least three months. These include weight reduction, increased exercise, reduced alcohol and salt intake and stopping smoking. Reduction of stresses and relaxation therapy helps, as does avoiding drugs which may cause hypertension, such as the oral contraceptive pill, non-steroidal anti-inflammatories and some antidepressants. Mild therapy involves the use of diuretics to increase the excretion of excess fluid, drugs targeting a specific part of the cardiovascular system, or combinations of these. Therapy should be monitored carefully. It is best to measure blood pressure first thing in the morning, before any medication is taken.

**HERBAL TREATMENT: Garlic,** one of the prime movers in lowering cholesterol and protecting against hypertension and heart disease; **celery seed,** particularly for its ability to encourage the excretion of excess fluid and as a circulatory tonic; **ginseng,** an antioxidant tonic; **psyllium,** to help lower blood cholesterol; **yarrow,** specifically for high blood pressure; **rosehip,** as a general circulatory tonic; **valerian,** in combination with other herbs.

**OTHER USEFUL NATURAL REMEDIES:** The best known supplement for hypertension is probably vitamin E; others include evening primrose oil, which lowers blood pressure and cholesterol, vitamin C with bioflavonoids, B-complex with added B3 and B6, and possibly minerals such as potassium and magnesium, which should be prescribed by a health practitioner if you are taking medication. The diet should be low in meat, fat and sugar, with no added salt and high in whole grains, fresh fruit, vegetables and oily fish. Gentle exercise and regular massage assist, and acupuncture may be helpful.

# IMMUNE SYSTEM

The immune system is the amazingly complex guardian of the body. Its job is to protect the body from infection and the development of any abnormal conditions, such as cancer. It has many components: the lymphatic vessels and lymph nodes; organs such as the tonsils, adrenals, spleen and thymus; the white blood cells; and antibodies and specialized cells. Its overall function is to protect "self" and eliminate "non-self." If the immune system is overwhelmed, infection or disease develop. If it falsely recognizes the "self" as a foreigner, one of the autoimmune diseases develops. The immune system is affected by our nutritional state and by our physical and psychological well-being.

In ancient times, many cultures believed that illness was caused by demons or evil spirits; some civilizations discovered earlier than others that physical things, rather than magical ones, could have been more important to health than previously believed, and began their search for a more scientific understanding of illnesses. The ancient Egyptians, for example, achieved a high degree of expertise in their methods of embalming, due to their medical and religious knowledge. This enabled modern medicine to have more of an understanding of some of the illnesses of the time. Even at that time, it is

obvious that garlic was regarded as a great body strengthener and protector; garlic cloves were found in the tomb of Tutankamen, dating from around 1352 B.C., as well as in tombs of many other pharaohs and common people. Records show that it was fed daily to the slaves who built the pyramids, to make sure their health was optimal. The Egyptians also saw the onion, now known to be a potent food that can reduce the length and severity of infections, as a powerful health strengthener; its layers representing heaven, earth and the nether world, and it, along with garlic, was widely used medicinally to strengthen the body. Perhaps it was at this time that physicians began to learn how to "strengthen the body," and therefore build up the body's immune system response.

**SYMPTOMS:** Our immune system responds to a challenge in a variety of ways. The response may be as simple as a fever, nausea, vomiting, swelling, redness, rash or fatigue; or as complex as diseases such as lupus, diabetes, rheumatoid arthritis, multiple sclerosis, psoriasis, HIV infection and cancer. Each of these must be looked at individually.

**TREATMENT:** The body can be protected through good nutritional support, the relief of stress factors and the creation of an environment of wellness. Vaccination is one approach to supporting the immune system, by priming it to deal with certain invaders. Antibiotics may be used to eliminate infectious agents. Other drugs either reduce our immune response and the specific disease that develops from it, or enhance our immune system's actions.

HERBAL TREATMENT: **Echinacea**, an excellent booster for the immune system; **garlic**, the antibiotic, antiviral, antibacterial protector; **gentian**, with its ability to raise the white cell count; **calendula**, widely used to stimulate the immune system and prevent infection; **ginkgo**, which has a free-radical scavenging effect; **St. John's wort**, with its anti-viral qualities; **ginseng**, an herb which can adapt to the body's needs; **licorice**, which contains protective estrogen-like compounds; **tea tree**, an immunostimulant.

OTHER USEFUL NATURAL REMEDIES: The most beneficial supplements are probably vitamin A; vitamin C with bioflavonoids; vitamins E and B-complex; a mineral compound tablet, particularly iron, zinc and magnesium; and possibly evening primrose oil.

Overall, developing a state of health within the body will allow it to have a strong, well-functioning immune system. Have sufficient rest, avoid coffee, alcohol and smoking, sleep well and eat wholesome foods. Stress reduction measures such as massage, aromatherapy, reflexology, meditation and regular exercise will also help strengthen the immune system.

Honey was also valued by the ancient Egyptians for its curative properties, and has now been found to have a solid basis in science, as clinical research has shown that certain disease producing micro-organisms cannot live in its presence. When placed in a culture of honey, the bacillus of typhoid fever died in less than 48 hours, while the pneumonia and bronchitis bacteria died after three days. Pure honey can assist in the removal of the environment which allows these bacteria to survive — it can be an invaluable assistant in helping to provide natural immunity for all sorts of conditions.

*The human body has two types of immunity – the first is a general form of defence that we are born with or that we acquire through our mother's milk. This is called Passive Immunity, and protects babies while they are developing their own immunity. The second is Acquired Immunity, which develops as we come in contact with new viruses and bacteria; our bodies can learn to "remember" previous viral or bacterial invaders and rapidly provide a quick defense against them.*

# INDIGESTION

Indigestion may be due to many disorders, including peptic ulceration, reflux of gastric acid or alkaline fluid, causing inflammation, ulceration, or even stricture of the esophagus, eating too quickly or eating too much, and eating rich or inadequately chewed food. Many drugs disturb the digestive system, such as aspirin, non-steroidal anti-inflammatories and steroids, as well as alcohol. Psychological factors such as stress and depression also play a part.

In ancient times, as now, indigestion was generally seen as a result of having too much of a good thing — and yet that didn't stop it happening; we've probably spent thousands of years working out how to cope with the after effects of the night before's indulgence, and sometimes, the long-term effects of ill-chosen foods. All ancient cultures have had remedies for indigestion, whether it was for the short-term effects of the night-before's meal, or longer term dietary inadequacies. In ancient Egypt, parsley was always added to meals to help alleviate the after-effects of the rich foods;

*"To eat every day, three to five fresh peas, or dried peas soaked in water, never cooked"*

OLD EUROPEAN REMEDY FOR INDIGESTION

and it is still used in modern times to help expel gas, for stomach aches, and to freshen breath.

The Chinese believed that the stomach helped control many emotions of the body; therefore anger, apprehension, over-excitement and other extreme emotions could affect the function of the stomach. Interestingly, Native American medicine closely followed the path of ancient Chinese medicine. Through their belief in attempting to understand the link between heaven and earth to understand health, they both developed herbs which could help maintain health, particularly in treating digestive disorders such as indigestion; their herbs may have been different, but the principles, and probably the active ingredients, were much the same.

In all probability, all around the world, all through time, healers have sought and found herbs which can help soothe the problems of the stomach, to help alleviate the many forms of indigestion caused by the many types of dietary lapses throughout civilization.

**SYMPTOMS:** Symptoms are most common after eating and are generally worse when bending or stooping. They include heartburn, nausea, upper abdominal pain often associated with bloating, flatulence and the mouth filling with saliva. There may be an association between reflux, asthma, nocturnal cough and bronchitis. Marked cases may have bleeding, associated anemia, and difficulty swallowing.

**TREATMENT:** Avoid irritants such as coffee, chocolate, fatty foods, spicy foods and alcohol. Eat frequent, small meals to keep the stomach contents neutralized, avoid heavy evening meals, eat slowly and not on the run. Weight reduction, elevating the head of the bed and loose clothing may help.

Stop smoking and try relaxation or stress management. Antacids are helpful to relieve symptoms, either in the form of a glass of milk, an antacid preparation or a mixture of antacid and alginate.

About 50 percent of people respond to these simple measures. More specific drugs help reduce gastric acid reduction. Other drugs such as metoclopramide help to empty the stomach more rapidly.

**HERBAL TREATMENT: Peppermint**, probably the best known remedy for indigestion; **meadowsweet**, a specific for peptic ulcers; **chamomile**, which improves appetite and relieves indigestion; **dandelion**, which assists the whole digestive system; **alfalfa**, the great alkalizer; **aloe vera** and **marshmallow**, for their soothing qualities; **gentian**, particularly for nausea, dyspepsia and stomach ulcers; **ginger**, particularly for an underactive digestion; **psyllium** and **slippery elm**, which soothe any inflammation or disturbance of the gastrointestinal tract; **ginseng**, particularly when indigestion is related to mental and nervous exhaustion and stress.

**OTHER USEFUL NATURAL REMEDIES:** Diet is one of the most important factors to consider.

Adding acidophilus yogurt to the daily wholefood regime is a good idea, and drinking several cups of peppermint and chamomile tea (separately) will also assist. Fennel is very helpful, especially for infants. Stress management techniques such as yoga, relaxation or meditation can be useful, as can homeopathy, acupuncture, reflexology and aromatherapy.

Russian folk medicine has long advocated potato therapy: raw, unpeeled, finely grated potatoes, with the juice; this should be puréed, with one cup taken three times a day before meals to avoid indigestion or other stomach complaints.

The ancient Egyptians used dill to treat indigestion, flatulence and colic; dill water is still used today for the same reasons, particularly for children with colic or as an ingredient in modern indigestion compounds.

*"If there be much tenderness, we may apply leeches over the stomach. With less tenderness, counter-irritation will answer – blisters, croton oil, mustard poultices, the compound tar plaster, or dry cups."*

MEDIEVAL REMEDY FOR INDIGESTION

# INFECTIONS

Considering that our world is one big playground for micro-organisms, we succumb to infection relatively rarely. We live in harmony with many organisms and call them our normal "flora." Our susceptibility to becoming infected depends on an organism's nature and on our defence mechanisms. The skin, the filtering system and mucus of our respiratory system, and our gastric acids all act as barriers. Our immune system is the army that deals with the invaders. Infections occur if the defense mechanism fails. Our defenses are reduced by poor sanitation, poor diet, stress and tension, drug therapy or pre-existing diseases.

Infections, of course, have been an established part of recorded history throughout all cultures and civilizations.

*An ancient remedy, which probably saved many thousands from amputation, is still used today: Take some black bread, such as rye or whole-grain, and cover it with salt. Chew it for a long time, until it is totally permeated with saliva. Then pack the masss tightly around the infected wound and bandage; this will stop the infection and prevent gangrene.*

Various forms of bacteria or germ have always been there to attack weakened tissue — infection, in most ancient times, was frequently a life-threatening condition, particularly in cultures where cleanliness and hygiene were not considered important or not believed to be of any relevance to the state of the body's health.

Many cultures, such as the Egyptians, did believe in cleanliness and hygiene, but more because they believed it was important to the gods, and therefore, they perhaps unknowingly helped ward off infections through their religious beliefs. Myrrh, for example, has strong biblical images as a precious substance, and yet the ancient Egyptian housewives burned it and anointed with it to cleanse and protect against evil spirits; today myrrh is still used to treat sore throats and respiratory infections. Garlic is another herb that has had widespread use through the ages to ward off infection, for both medicinal and religious reasons, as have many other herbs, now shown to be effective scientifically.

**SYMPTOMS:** Fever — an elevation of the body temperature above its normal — is the hallmark of infection. This can be accompanied by an increased heart rate, respiratory rate and, at times, anxiety, confusion and even delirium. When we are infected, white cells usually multiply, a blood test will confirm this. Then there are the signs relating to whichever system is infected, such as a cough for the respiratory system, pus in the skin and so on.

TREATMENT: Creating a strong body both externally and internally reduces the chances of any organisms taking hold. Many infections are mild and self-limiting, so general principles are the most important, such as treat the fever, maintain a nourishing diet, take plenty of fluids, and support with nursing care.

There are three possible outcomes to infection:

• The defense mechanisms eradicate the organism (or extra treatment is required, such as antibiotics) and the host returns to a normal state with a specific protective immunity developed.

• A state of equilibrium is achieved and chronic infection occurs.

• The organisms multiply and the host dies.

Antibiotics play a vital role when the evidence points to an organism which would be susceptible to them. Preventative measures aim at stopping the infection's spread from one person to another. If you have an infection, it is important to protect others from contact with your bodily fluids, so always cover your face if you cough, wash your hands, avoid contact with blood and stools, and so on.

Vaccines may be given to induce an immune response and prevent subsequent disease. This is a controversial area, however. Vaccines can be considered a major public health benefit but they carry risks as well as advantages. No vaccine is completely safe or completely effective.

HERBAL TREATMENT: **Echinacea** and **garlic**, the magnificent herbal antibiotics; **tea tree**, a powerful immunostimulant; **thyme**, with its strong antiseptic action, and **ginseng** in the recovery period, are probably the most effective, although many other herbs can be beneficial.

OTHER USEFUL NATURAL REMEDIES: Vitamins C, A, E and B-complex, as well as zinc, calcium, magnesium and iron help deal with the stress of the infection and assist our natural resistance. Acidophilus/lactobacillus yogurt or tablets help restore the natural bacteria of the intestines. Drink plenty of water, eat fresh fruit and vegetables, and rest.

Many other herbs have been used since ancient times to help treat infections. Native Americans, for example, traditionally used chapparal, yucca and golden seal for all infections or toxic conditions.

For a local infection of the skin, try applying a combination of calendula, comfrey and St. John's wort ointments twice daily — this combination will assist in reducing infection, assisting healing, and reducing inflammation and pain.

*In Tibet, healers still open an infected wound and smear it with an animal's fresh blood daily.*

# INFLUENZA

This common viral respiratory tract infection occurs mostly in winter. It is spread by droplets, so every time an infected person breathes out, sneezes, laughs, coughs or talks, people nearby are liable to become infected.

Influenza is caused by a multitude of viruses and epidemics may sporadically erupt. These viruses can change their nature to fool our immune systems. Incubation is approximately 48 hours. Influenza A causes the worldwide epidemics during which 10–40 percent of a population may be affected. Influenzas B and C are less dangerous.

**SYMPTOMS:** The clinical picture varies with a person's age. It ranges from presenting with a slight fever to a combination of fever, headache, harsh dry cough, muscle ache (especially lower back and legs), dry sore throat and pain behind the sternum. Croup is common in children under five. Children may also have convulsions, vomiting and painful sensitivity to strong light. In the elderly, the symptoms of more severe disease, such as pneumonia, usually do not show up until late in the illness.

**TREATMENT:** Influenza usually lasts from four to seven days, although sometimes people experience a second wave of symptoms. Most treatment is supportive — bed rest, good fluid intake and an agent that reduces fever, such as paracetamol. Antibiotics only have a role if secondary bacterial infection is present. Complications include pneumonia, middle ear infection, sinusitis, encephalitis and myocarditis.

Prevention by pre-winter vaccination is recommended for at-risk people, especially those with chronic heart or lung problems, or chronic diseases such as diabetes or kidney failure. People over 65 years and those in care facilities should also be covered.

The drug amantadine is useful for people exposed to influenza A to prevent and shorten the illness. In uncomplicated cases, rapid recovery is the rule.

**HERBAL TREATMENT:** A large number of herbs are helpful in reducing symptoms, including **garlic**, **echinacea**, **yarrow**, **tea tree**, **thyme**, **chamomile**, **rosehip**, **ginger**, **elder flower**, **licorice** and **ginseng**.

**OTHER USEFUL NATURAL REMEDIES:** It is most important to build up the immune system, so take vitamins A, B, C and E, plus zinc. Drink fluids frequently, avoid rich, highly processed or fatty foods, alcohol and coffee, eat small meals of fresh fruit, vegetables or soup, and get as much rest as possible. Herbal inhalants and oils such as tea tree or eucalyptus in an oil burner or rubbed on the chest may help.

# INSOMNIA

We all need different amounts of sleep for a sense of well-being and refreshment the next morning. The amount we need usually diminishes with age. This is a physiological change, but some elderly people become so disturbed about their lack of sleep that they experience further insomnia. People often overestimate their periods of sleeplessness. Causes of insomnia include pain, anxiety, depression, rebound after the use of sedatives, alcohol or drugs, sleep apnoea (episodes of stopping breathing in sleep), heart failure, restless leg syndrome, medications (for example, asthma treatment, diet tablets, antidepressants), and time phase alteration in shift workers or following long plane trips.

**SYMPTOMS:** Insomnia is characterized by difficulty in falling and remaining asleep, frequent night wakening, lack of restful sleep, early morning final awakening, or a combination of these. There is often associated depression, anxiety or drug and alcohol use.

**TREATMENT:** The most suitable treatment is often established with a knowledge of the history. It is important to treat the underlying condition, especially pain. What is tolerable during the day is often intolerable at night.

Keeping a sleep chart to assess the sleeping–waking cycle is useful. Medication should be used for the shortest possible time and in the lowest dose, as it may give undesirable side effects the next day.

Drugs can be targeted as sleep inducers or sleep maintainers. Marked sedative action can be provided by antidepressants. The newest form of sleep therapy is the hypnotic zopiclone which increases the quality and length of sleep but does not reduce REM (rapid eye movement or dream sleep). All these medications are open to abuse. Going to a sleep laboratory for assessment can be helpful if there is a long history of insomnia or a failure to respond to treatment.

**HERBAL TREATMENT:** The most effective herbal helpers are **valerian**, the modern-day tranquilizer and **chamomile**, the gentle soother. Many other herbs may assist, but it is best to have a specific prescription made up for you if the problem is chronic.

**OTHER USEFUL NATURAL REMEDIES:** Simple measures are to avoid alcohol, coffee, tea and chocolate later in the evening and decrease smoking, eating and exercise prior to retiring.

Adopting a lifestyle which helps to promote sleep is essential. It is helpful to take regular exercise (but not at bedtime) and have a personal bedtime routine with a reduction of noise and other distractions. Behavior modification with relaxation, hypnosis, meditation or biofeedback may enable a gradual return to biological rhythms. Vitamin B3 and B6 taken an hour before bed with a "sleepytime" herbal tea may help.

# LIVER DISORDERS

The liver, one of the largest organs in the body, is the metabolic powerhouse, with more than 500 identified functions. It produces substances such as bile and proteins, it metabolizes our foods, it detoxifies the blood of unwanted hormones, chemicals and toxins (alcohol is a well-known example) and produces and stores glycogen which regulates the body's energy supply. The best recognized disorders are hepatitis, cirrhosis and tumors, with jaundice a common sign.

Cirrhosis is characterized by death of the liver cells and replacement with scar tissue. Hepatitis is inflammation of the liver by a virus or by a toxin e.g. alcohol. As all the blood in the body flows through and is filtered by the liver, this is a common site for secondary cancers (and also primary ones, that is, cancers that start in the liver).

Disorders of the liver can manifest in all parts of the body, and can include such varied symptoms as fatigue, weakened muscles, food intolerance, acne, nausea and bowel dysfuntion (either diarrhea, constipation or flatulence). The liver, unlike most organs, does have regenerative abilities, but needs substantial help in the form of rest, correct diet, and abstinence from aggravating factors (toxins) to be able to heal itself. When it is overloaded, the liver is unable to fulfill its major function of detoxifying the blood, which can lead to toxicity problems and many general ill-health conditions. Even overeating has been known to create fatty deposits within the liver, and this can lead to an overworked and enlarged organ struggling to function at its best.

The liver has long been considered one of the most important body organs in traditional Chinese medicine. It is associated with the emotion of suppressed anger and the lack of the "wood" element, which shows as a slow morning riser and general irritability.

**SYMPTOMS:** Jaundice is one of the major signs of liver disease, but it can also be caused by the breakdown of blood cells or a blockage (for example, from gallstones). There is yellowness of the whites of the eyes, the skin and the mucous membranes. Urine goes dark and the stools go pale. Fatigue, itchiness, liver discomfort, nausea, vomiting and fever may all be part of liver disease.

A number of symptoms may indicate liver sluggishness, which makes it difficult to diagnose; these include fatigue (especially after meals), a feeling of fullness or tenderness below the right ribs, headaches, constipation or diarrhea or both, flatulence and digestion problems, bad breath and skin problems.

**TREATMENT:** Given the many causes of assault on the liver, there are many directions of treatment. General supportive measures of rest, good fluid intake and a well-balanced and nutritious diet are important, with small low-fat, low-protein, high-carbohydrate meals. Alcohol or other suspected toxins are best avoided.

Associated symptoms of nausea or itchiness should be treated.

If an infection is responsible it is important to trace all contacts, protect them, and treat them where necessary, and make them aware of how the infection can be spread. Interferon has been used in the treatment of Hepatitis C. Liver transplant may be the only option with advanced cirrhosis.

**HERBAL TREATMENT:** There are quite a few powerful liver herbs, in particular: **dandelion**, frequently used for jaundice, hepatitis and in the early stages of cirrhosis; **milk thistle**, also for jaundice and stimulating bile flow; **garlic**, which regulates liver function; **devil's claw**, a liver cleanser and detoxifier; **senna**, when associated with constipation; **echinacea**, for its action against invading viruses and bacteria; **gentian**, as it increases bile flow, assists jaundice and biliousness; **ginseng**, for its stimulating qualities; **licorice** and **rosemary**, for a sluggish liver, and **yarrow**, for impaired liver function of nervous origin.

**OTHER USEFUL NATURAL REMEDIES:** Diet is particularly important when any abnormal liver condition occurs. Apart from avoiding fats, highly refined foods, as many chemicals as possible and excess sugar and alcohol, try adding red beet juice, grape juice, lemon juice and brewer's yeast to the diet. The B-complex vitamins are probably the most important supplement (brewer's yeast is a good source) as well as high doses of vitamin C, betacarotene and zinc. Dandelion coffee is helpful.

Shiatsu may be particularly beneficial — in this ancient Japanese system of healing, the liver is more important than any other organ, as it is believed to ensure the flow of chi, or life force, through the whole body. Acupressure and acupuncture are also extremely beneficial, and several of Dr. Bach's flower remedies may assist with the underlying emotions involved with liver conditions. Aromatherapy treatments, particularly with the use of the essential oils of rosemary, peppermint and chamomile, may also greatly assist — these oils stimulate the production of bile and act as general liver tonics, and may be also added to hot compresses applied over the liver area.

*"The liver is ruler over the spring. It is the root of life's ultimate action; its condition is revealed in the fingernails and toenails as well as in the muscles."*

CHINESE FOLK MEDICINE

141

# MENSTRUAL DISCOMFORT

Most women experience some degree of period pain, or dysmenorrhea, at some time, ranging from a slight dragging sensation to extreme pain. It may begin in their teens, shortly after the onset of menstruation. This is known as primary or spasmodic dysmenorrhea and is due to uterine contractions, hormonal imbalance or psychological factors, such as anxiety about periods. Secondary dysmenorrhea is the result of pelvic disease, such as pelvic inflammatory disease, endometriosis, fibroids, ovarian cysts or pelvic tumors. Other factors involved are an increase in the level of prostaglandins which produce muscle spasms, and menstrual clots which may obstruct flow and cause pressure and pain.

**SYMPTOMS:** Primary dysmenorrhea causes pain at the onset of, or just before, the period. It lasts from a few hours to one day or more. Cramping occurs in the lower abdomen, lower back and legs. There may be nausea, vomiting, loose stools or even fainting. Secondary dysmenorrhea begins several days before the period and can last for the entire time of bleeding. There is a dull, aching pain in the lower abdomen. Other symptoms are dizziness, depression, painful bladder or bowel function, headache, backache, abdominal distension and pain on intercourse.

**TREATMENT:** It is important to distinguish between primary and secondary dysmenorrhea. A pelvic examination is usually necessary to rule out abnormalities in the pelvis. In primary dysmenorrhea, simple analgesics may be all that is needed. Non-steroidal anti-inflammatories may also reduce the pain. The oral contraceptive pill (preferably low dose) to prevent ovulation or progesterone treatment will help. Surgical treatment to dilate the cervix was once commonly done and gives temporary relief, but is now only used, together with curette and laparoscopy, as part of diagnosis. In secondary dysmenorrhea the treatment depends on the underlying cause: antibiotics for infections, hormone therapy for endometriosis, dilation of the canal in cervical narrowing; and surgery for uterine malformations, fibroids or endometriosis. Primary dysmenorrhea often ends with the first pregnancy.

**HERBAL TREATMENT:** Many herbs may assist with this condition, depending on the presenting symptoms. They include **chamomile**, **valerian**, **yarrow**, **willow bark**, **ginger**, **alfalfa**, **raspberry leaf**, **marshmallow**, **calendula**, **thyme** and **psyllium**.

**OTHER USEFUL NATURAL REMEDIES:** Evening primrose oil, vitamin E, B-complex vitamins, iron and magnesium may all be of assistance. Adequate sleep, rest and exercise are important. Yoga is helpful for stretching and relaxing muscles and improving the circulation. A hot water bottle or a bath is often the best therapy.

# MIGRAINES

One of the most severe headaches, migraines are unfortunately also extremely common. They usually start in childhood, adolescence, at the menopause, with the use of the oral contraceptive pill and in pregnancy. Most patients give a positive family history. Migraines are the result of the dilation and then contraction of blood vessels of the head.

**SYMPTOMS:** Classical migraines last from two to 72 hours. The intense headache is usually on one side of the head and accompanied by nausea, vomiting and a painful sensitivity to light. There can be specific neurological changes, for example, weakness in a limb or change in vision, but these usually fade away. Many patients experience forewarning in the form of visual disturbance. Cluster migraines last a few hours or present daily; they can go on for months and then disappear, sometimes returning. They usually occur behind one eye with associated runny eye, nose and swollen red face on the affected side.

**TREATMENT:** Migraines developing for the first time in middle age, especially if there is no family history, must be investigated. They may be triggered by foods, such as chocolate, caffeine, citrus fruits, cheese, alcohol (especially red wine), MSG, food preservatives and drugs, such as estrogen or the combined oral contraceptive pill. Other triggers are emotional stress (the most common) or physical stress (for example, exercise), heat, bright lights, dry winds and menstruation. So if you can identify any trigger and avoid it, this will help. Treatment is usually simple analgesics, and if given early enough they may abort the attack.

If at least two severe migraine attacks occur per month then prophylactic therapy is important. This may include the prescription of antiseratonin or antihistamine agents, such as pizotifen or methysergide, beta-blockers or antidepressants. Probably the most effective treatment is learning how to manage tension and stress and using relaxation exercises.

**HERBAL TREATMENT: Feverfew** is the most effective herbal preventative for migraine; **willow bark**, **meadowsweet**, **valerian** and **devil's claw** may be of assistance for their analgesic, anti-inflammatory effects; other herbs may be indicated, depending upon the particular symptoms.

**OTHER USEFUL NATURAL REMEDIES:** It is wise to try to eliminate any possible food triggers from the diet, and eat regular, well-balanced meals (low blood sugar can sometimes trigger a migraine, so avoid missing meals). Adding vitamin and mineral supplements may help, as well as regular massage, aromatherapy or reflexology treatments. Homeopathy and acupuncture may be helpful, as well as yoga or meditation. Lying quietly in a darkened room with a cold compress on the head, sipping yarrow tea, with lavender, rosemary or chamomile essential oil in an oil burner may provide relief.

# MOTION SICKNESS

Motion sickness is easier to avoid than to treat. Repetitive stimulation of our inner ear mechanism (the labyrinth) sends messages to the brain's vomiting center. It is typically brought on by any movement which has repetitive acceleration and deceleration and is accentuated by stimuli such as smells (fumes or smoke), poor ventilation, emotion (fear), or visual stimuli (such as a moving horizon).

**SYMPTOMS:** Prior to its onset there is often increased salivation, yawning, sleepiness or profuse sweating. The nausea and vomiting occur in waves and may be accompanied by headache, vertigo and poor concentration. A steady horizon and fresh air may settle symptoms. Prolonged vomiting is a great stress on the body, and may cause dehydration and lowered blood pressure, so make sure that in recovery there's a high fluid intake.

**TREATMENT:** An ounce of prevention is worth a bucket of cure. Prophylactic drugs given before exposure to the motion can help. These include antihistamines, orally or by injection, and skin patches. Sedatives and anxiety-relieving medications may help. If vomiting is established then antinausea preparations may be useful, as well as maintaining the hydration of the patient. Acupressure points (such as between the thumb and forefinger) can be manipulated during a journey to help relieve the nausea.

**HERBAL TREATMENT: Ginger** is the specific remedy for motion sickness; **alfalfa**, **gentian**, **milk thistle** and **peppermint** can also assist, as can the relaxing and calming effects of **valerian** and **chamomile**.

**OTHER USEFUL NATURAL REMEDIES:** Physical adjustments are useful. When traveling, don't read; stay in a well-ventilated space; ride in the front of the car (reclining or lying down with a head support); avoid alcohol; have small, frequent meals; and try to look above the horizon rather than at moving objects. Taking vitamin B6 daily may also help.

*Motion sickness includes air sickness, car sickness, sickness on rides or swings, and sea sickness (sometimes known as* mal de mer).

# NAUSEA

When nausea occurs the stomach slows down its normal emptying and the duodenum (the part of the digestive tract just below the stomach) tightens, sometimes forcing its contents back into the stomach. Then we have the sensation of retching, and if this continues we will vomit. This is brought about by messages from the vomiting center of the brain. There are a multitude of causes. It can be related to the abdomen (for example ulcer, obstruction), infections, the brain (for example increased pressure, tumor), the inner ear, or labyrinth (for example motion sickness), systemic diseases (for example diabetes, gall bladder disease), thyroid disease, early pregnancy, drugs (for example alcohol, toxins, therapeutic drugs and drug withdrawal). Nausea can also arise from psychological causes, such as anxiety, anorexia and bulimia.

**SYMPTOMS:** Nausea is the sensation that you wish to vomit, often felt in the throat or upper abdomen. There may be accompanying waterbrash (fluid coming up into the mouth), consisting of mucus and saliva and contractions of the abdomen. We may or may not be able to stop the next step — vomiting. If the symptoms are persistent or severe, seek medical advice.

**TREATMENT:** Look for the cause and treat this first. Nausea is a very common symptom for a range of conditions from mild ones to those that are life threatening. Try eating and drinking in small amounts and stick to light foods, such as biscuits, pasta, soup and rice. Avoid fatty foods. Sometimes flat soft drinks help or honey in water. Avoid getting hungry. Replace fluid lost if there is vomiting.

There are several medications to relieve nausea. The well-known antiemetics are prochlorperazine and metoclopramide, which act on the vomiting center. Antihistamines are also useful. In the nausea of pregnancy drugs must be used with care.

**HERBAL TREATMENT: Ginger** is one of the most effective antinausea herbs. Others include **alfalfa**, which alkalizes the system; **peppermint** and **chamomile**, which are relaxing to the stomach and antispasmodic; **meadowsweet**, which normalizes stomach function; **devil's claw**, a useful anti-inflammatory; **gentian**, a tonic for the whole digestive system; **ginseng**, particularly when associated with mental or nervous stress; **marshmallow**, for its soothing effects; **psyllium**, rich in mucilage; **raspberry leaf**, particularly in pregnancy, and many other herbs.

**OTHER USEFUL NATURAL REMEDIES:** Stay with a simple, light, fat-free diet, to which acidophilus yogurt and slippery elm powder have been added. Have frequent small sips of water (but not cold water), dill water, ginger or chamomile tea to prevent dehydration. A vitamin B6 supplement may assist, but if symptoms persist, see a medical practitioner.

# POSTURAL HYPOTENSION

Postural hypotension refers to the response that some people have when they move from lying down, sitting or kneeling to standing. Their blood pressure falls and they suffer associated symptoms.

We normally maintain our blood pressure through a central controlling system — another one of those amazing feats of body physiology of which we are blissfully unaware. This system receives information from pressure-sensing elements in our cardiovascular system. If this system fails, we cannot adjust the blood pressure to postural change, or we do it too slowly. There are many causes, including heart disease, a defect in the nervous system that occurs in old age, certain drugs, excessive alcohol use, Parkinson's disease, diabetes mellitus, anemia, varicose veins and excessive sweating.

**SYMPTOMS:** Often symptoms are minor and vague, but the relationship to the change in posture is the important factor. They may also be brought on by exercise or a heavy meal.

Symptoms are usually transient and include blurred vision, nausea, dizziness and light-headedness. Occasionally there can be more severe effects such as sudden collapse and unconsciousness, even generalized seizures.

**TREATMENT:** First of all, it is important to eliminate any obvious causes. Drugs, especially overzealous treatment of the elderly with cardiovascular disease, may be responsible. Adequate hydration must be maintained. Correcting these usually fixes the problem.

Increasing the sodium intake can be effective. Make sure food is well salted or take salt tablets. This change in diet may need an accompanying increase in potassium by way of a supplement or by diet, such as eating bananas. Stimulating the system with adrenalin (ephedrine) during waking hours may also help.

Care in the change of posture is probably the most important feature. Move to an upright position slowly and avoid prolonged standing.

**HERBAL TREATMENT:** A number of different herbs are useful in treating this condition. It is a good idea to boost the functioning of the circulatory system with such herbs as **ginkgo**, **yarrow**, **alfalfa**, **dandelion**, **garlic**, **celery**, **rosehip** or **devil's claw**. Others may also be indicated, depending on the individual symptom picture.

**OTHER USEFUL NATURAL REMEDIES:** The best advice is to make sure your diet is as healthy as possible: avoid highly processed, fatty foods, eat whole grains, fruits and vegetables, drink fluids regularly, and exercise gently every day. Yoga, massage, reflexology and acupuncture may assist. General supplements should include vitamins A, C, E, B-complex and a multimineral tablet.

# PREMENSTRUAL SYNDROME

## (PMS)

This is a collection of symptoms, usually occurring for 7 to 10 days before menstruation begins. It tends to be more severe after age twenty-five. The cause is unclear but has been related to variations in the levels of estrogen and progesterone hormones, with estrogen causing fluid retention. Other causes may be related to nutritional deficiencies, various emotional disorders or changes in glands such as the adrenals.

**SYMPTOMS:** Emotional instability occurs, ranging from depression to anxiety. Headaches (including the exacerbation of migraines), fatigue, insomnia, lower back pain, acne, breast pain, lower abdominal bloating, weight gain (which is lost after menstruation begins), ankle edema (fluid retention in the ankle), food cravings, difficulty concentrating, lack of co-ordination and lack of libido may all be part of the picture. A few or all of these may occur.

**TREATMENT:** If the symptoms are mild, reassurance that PMS is a natural occurrence may be the best treatment. Otherwise, whatever symptoms there are should be treated. Understanding is an important step to solving the problem. Sometimes mild diuretics are used but a traditional approach is to increase fluid intake to make the kidneys work better. Analgesics or antidepressants may be needed. A bra with good support will provide relief from breast pain. Counseling may be necessary. Hormone therapy using progesterone can assist.

Improving the diet helps reduce fluid retention and other symptoms. Avoid salt, tea, coffee, alcohol and cocoa products (such as chocolate), do not smoke, and increase intake of whole grains, fruits and vegetables.

**HERBAL TREATMENT: Alfalfa** and **licorice**, hormonal herbs with estrogen mimicking qualities; **celery**, for its diuretic properties; **raspberry leaf**, commonly used for all sorts of female conditions; **licorice**, for general "feeling low" symptoms; **chamomile**, for its gentle, relaxing qualities.

**OTHER USEFUL NATURAL REMEDIES:** Valuable supplements include vitamins B1 and B6 as well as a B-complex and mineral compound tablet (including iron, zinc and magnesium), regular vitamins C and E, and evening primrose oil. Aromatherapy, massage, reflexology, Dr. Bach's Flower Remedies, homeopathy and acupuncture may all be beneficial.

# SCIATICA

This is one of the most common back problems. It is caused by irritation or pressure on the sciatic nerve roots, usually due to a prolapsed intervertebral disc, disc degeneration or osteoarthritis. More rarely it is due to a spinal tumor or ankylosing spondylitis, a disease that causes chronic inflammation of the spine and adjacent skeletal structures, which may cause fusion of the spine. It may be exacerbated by pregnancy.

**SYMPTOMS:** Pain may be either a dull, continuous ache or severe, sharp and shooting — enough to put you to bed. The pain follows part or all of the nerve pathway, that is, from lower back to buttock, to back of thigh and then to the outside of the leg and ankle. Rest relieves the pain, but movement, especially forward bending, exercise, coughing, sneezing and straining make it worse. Severe cases will involve change or loss of sensation and muscle weakness, and loss of normal reflexes in the leg.

**TREATMENT:** The best treatment is to stay in bed with boards under the mattress, or pull the mattress on the floor and lie with hips and knees bent. Only get up to go to the toilet or to have hot baths or showers. Aspirin-based analgesics can ease the pain. Local heat and non-steroidal anti-inflammatories or muscle relaxants such as diazepam also help. Physiotherapy, osteopathy and massage are useful in relieving spasms in the surrounding muscles in the back and will help strengthen them. Learn to avoid those activities that bring sciatica on. A lumbosacral corset may help relieve chronic pain. In severe cases it might be necessary to perform surgery to relieve the pressure on the nerve.

**HERBAL TREATMENT: St. John's wort**, a potent helper for any nerve pain; **calendula**, **horse chestnut**, **thyme** and **devil's claw**, for their anti-inflammatory properties; **alfalfa**, as it helps eliminate excess uric acid; **gentian**, a tonic and antispasmodic; **willow bark**, **chamomile** and **valerian**, for their analgesic properties.

**OTHER USEFUL NATURAL REMEDIES:** The aim is to strengthen the nervous system as much as possible, so take B-complex vitamins or brewer's yeast and a mineral supplement on a regular basis. Daily, gentle strengthening exercises, such as stretching or yoga, can have long-term benefits. Regular massage, reflexology and acupuncture may also assist. In an acute situation, alternating hot and cold packs on the base of the spine, and then applying rue ointment or thyme oil, may bring relief.

# SKIN INFECTIONS

Skin infections are commonly caused by strains of the *Staphylococcus aureus* bacteria. Damaged skin or a weakened immune system can cause the body to be more susceptible to skin infections. "Golden Staph" is one of humanity's most significant pathogens. There seems to be an increasing incidence of antibiotic resistance to these bacteria and a multiresistant variety is often found in hospitals.

**SYMPTOMS:** *Boils* are nodules of pus that develop in a skin follicle and are often extremely tender. They tend to be recurrent and are frequently found on the buttocks, armpits, breasts, face and neck. *Carbuncles* develop more slowly, occur in clusters, go deep and have multiple openings for the discharge of pus. They heal slowly, leave scars, and are commonly found on the nape of the neck. They are more frequently found in males, diabetics, the elderly and the seriously ill. *Folliculitis* is a redness, a pustule or nodule around a hair follicle. *Impetigo* is a blistering, pussy skin condition that is mostly found in children. It occurs on the face, hands and knees, and is characterized by a thick, yellowish crust and there are often multiple spots occurring in different stages of development.

**TREATMENT:** Prompt treatment is needed to avoid chronic infection, so always cleanse skin with antiseptic soap and wash towels, sheets and clothing in hot water. These conditions can be very contagious so wash your hands thoroughly after any contact. Antiseptics or antibiotic creams may be useful. A single boil may be able to come to the surface (point) and discharge its contents by applying hot packs. If the face is involved or the case is severe, oral antibiotics such as penicillin may be prescribed.

**HERBAL TREATMENT:** Depending on the condition, these may include eliminative herbs to aid the bloodstream, kidneys and digestion, such as **echinacea, garlic, yarrow, chamomile, dandelion, slippery elm, thyme, celery seed, milk thistle, St. John's wort** and **psyllium**. Vulnerary herbs (wound healers) include **tea tree, aloe vera, calendula, elder flower, marshmallow, witch hazel** and **yarrow** used externally.

**OTHER USEFUL NATURAL REMEDIES:** Build up the defense system with vitamin C. Flaxseed (linseed) poultices or cool arnica or stinging nettle compresses may assist if there is marked inflammation, and ointments, such as cowbane, marshmallow, tea tree and golden seal, may help greatly. Ensure the diet is high in fruits, vegetables and fiber. Many vitamin and mineral supplements may assist, but are best prescribed for each individual case. Drink plenty of fluids, exercise regularly, and see your naturopathic practitioner if the condition persists.

# STOMACH ULCERS

Stomach or peptic ulcer disease is common — 10 to 20 percent of people develop it in their lifetime. Ulcers may be in the stomach (gastric ulcer) or in the duodenum. They are essentially caused by an imbalance between the effect of acid pepsin in the gastric juices and the resistance of the mucous membranes to this. Factors which cause or prolong ulcers include cigarette smoking, genetic factors, drugs such as aspirin, non-steroidal anti-inflammatories and steroids, psychological stress, diet, alcohol, and the organism *Helicobacter pylori*.

**SYMPTOMS:** The most consistent symptom is a burning or gnawing pain, usually in the upper abdomen but sometimes in the back. It occurs one to two hours after meals and may wake the sufferer in the early hours of the morning. It can be relieved by food or antacids. There can be weight loss or gain. Nausea and vomiting occurs, and there can be blood in the vomit or stools which can be black and tarry.

**TREATMENT:** The aim of treatment is to relieve the symptoms, help healing of the ulcer and prevent recurrences. Eradication of *Helicobacter pylori* is important because the rate of recurrence becomes dramatically lower. This is done by "triple therapy":

treating with a combination of antibiotics and acid-lowering medications. Adjunctive therapy includes medicines that reduce the acid secretions. These medications give healing of more than 90 percent in eight weeks and reduce recurrences with long-term therapy.

Coating the ulcer surface helps protect it from the action of acid. Antacids (liquids are better than tablets) neutralize the acid but have to be taken frequently. About one-fifth of patients ultimately, because of complications, require surgery — either removal of the part of the stomach or duodenum affected by the ulcer, or cutting the vagus nerve that produces acid.

**HERBAL TREATMENT:** Quite a few herbs are invaluable for this condition, including **alfalfa**, **calendula**, **garlic**, **gentian**, **ginseng**, **licorice**, **marshmallow**, **meadowsweet** (specifically for peptic ulcers), **peppermint**, **psyllium** and **slippery elm**.

**OTHER USEFUL NATURAL REMEDIES:** General measures such as rest, stopping smoking, avoiding caffeine and alcohol help. Milk is frequently recommended, but the benefits are questionable. It is probably better to take chamomile tea. Bedtime snacks are best avoided but eating small, frequent meals may help. Avoid hot, spicy, highly processed or acidic foods. Relaxation techniques and stress control may assist. Other helpful treatments include Dr. Bach's Flower Remedies and homeopathy.

# STRESS

We commonly experience stress in our action-packed modern-day lives. The demands (or stressors) of job, lifestyle, family, finances and deadlines can accumulate to a point where we find it impossible to cope. Our environment also places stressors on us, including exposure to chemicals, toxins, even extremes of hot and cold weather, or physical injuries. It is not surprising that many of our modern ailments have stress as a contributing factor.

**SYMPTOMS:** The stressors of life can affect us in many ways. We experience any number of symptoms, including headaches, fatigue, an inability to concentrate, dyspepsia, ulcers, allergies, depression, anxiety, high blood pressure, high cholesterol levels, heart disease, adult onset diabetes, irritable bowel syndrome, ulcerative colitis, menstrual irregularities, premenstrual syndrome and rheumatoid arthritis.

**TREATMENT:** Anyone affected by stress needs to develop an individual strategy to manage that stress, not just to cope with it. It is best to attempt simple, lifestyle management techniques first, if you realize you are not coping. Exercise is important, but avoid competitive exercise as that just leads to additional stress. Try a walk around the block or in the park two or three times a week and take time to smell the roses.

Antidepressants, antianxiety preparations and hypnotics may be helpful if the condition becomes unmanageable, or leads to other stress-induced conditions.

**HERBAL TREATMENT:** Many herbs assist with the day-to-day stresses we face, including **chamomile**, which contains the amino acid tryptophan, a natural sedative; **dandelion**, rich in easily assimilated vitamin complexes and minerals and a major help in detoxifying the body; **echinacea** and **garlic**, which boost the immune system and help strengthen the whole body; **ginkgo**, which stimulates blood flow, particularly to the brain; **ginseng**, a whole-body tonic and restorative; **licorice**, an excellent herb to support the adrenal glands; **rosehip**, an invaluable vitamin C-rich tonic.

**OTHER USEFUL NATURAL REMEDIES:** To assist our body with everyday stressors we particularly need vitamin B-complex, vitamin C, zinc, potassium and magnesium. Eat a healthy, whole-food diet, with foods high in potassium and low in sodium, such as avocado, carrots, corn, potatoes, tomatoes, spinach, apples, apricots, bananas, oranges, strawberries and plums. Brewer's yeast, high in the B vitamins, is a good dietary supplement. Relaxation, tai chi, meditation, Dr. Bach's Flower Remedies, massage, aromatherapy and just taking time out will all help you manage stress.

# TEETH PROBLEMS

The teeth are made of modified bone but are considered part of our digestive system. They have two to four roots, each with their own blood supply and nerves. We have 20 childhood teeth and 32 permanent ones. Teeth may have a variety of conditions themselves, or they may be the underlying cause for face, head and neck pain. Tooth problems include decay (an extremely common problem), abscess and poor alignment.

Dental care is also extremely important in many systemic disorders (e.g. cancer), when taking various drugs which can reduce response to infection, in bleeding disorders, in leukemia, with heart valve disease, in diabetes, and with bulimia.

**SYMPTOMS:** Tooth decay generally causes no symptoms until well established, then there may be pain, especially after eating sugary foods, and sensitivity to hot and cold. Abscesses or inflammation of the dental pulp (the soft, spongy substance within the tooth) can cause sharp, throbbing or gnawing pain, and it may be difficult to bring the teeth together because of pain.

**TREATMENT:** Teeth problems may be related to an underlying systemic disease. Brushing teeth to remove food, plaque (a thin film on the teeth that harbors bacteria) and tartar (an encrustation deposited by the saliva) is essential. Try to avoid tooth grinding by retraining or wearing a mouthguard which is made specifically to fit your mouth by a dentist.

Always treat *gingivitis* (see page 125). *Tooth decay* requires restoration by dental fillings. Treatment with topical fluoride helps prevent tooth decay and chlorhexidine mouthwashes can help.

Treat *abcesses* by rinsing with hot, salty water to bring to a point. Abscesses usually require drainage by a dentist. Antibiotics may be necessary for treating abscesses. Analgesics are often needed to ease the pain of an abscess. Bed rest, soft-food diet, and lots of fluids help.

**HERBAL TREATMENT: Willow bark, chamomile** and **valerian** may help short term with toothache; **echinacea** and **garlic** can be taken for infection; **tea tree** and **thyme**, as an antiseptic mouthwash; **yarrow** and **calendula** for abscesses.

**OTHER USEFUL NATURAL REMEDIES:** Oil of cloves and tea tree oil can be applied to a tooth to relieve toothache. High doses of vitamin C and mineral supplements may also help.

# VARICOSE VEINS

We all have seen legs with dilated, tortuous veins and lumpy incompetent valves. The vein walls become thickened and nutrition to the leg becomes poor as a result of sluggish blood flow. If you happen to be a woman, elderly, unusually tall, have a family history or a job that requires prolonged standing, you have a greater chance of getting them. A rise in blood pressure in the leg veins from a deep venous thrombosis or pressure in the abdomen from pregnancy or tumors may also cause them. Recent studies suggest that the vein wall may have an inherent weakness in some people. Other sites for varicose veins are the scrotum, vulva and rectum. Those in the rectum are known as hemorrhoids.

**SYMPTOMS:** Symptoms include aching in the legs, heaviness (worse on standing and relieved by elevation), fatigue, itchiness of the legs, and swelling in the ankles. Later there is discoloration, broken capillaries, dermatitis, cellulitis and ulceration in the lower leg. The thin vein walls can blow out and rupture, causing hemorrhage, with little or no injury.

**TREATMENT:** Firstly, it is important to make sure that there is not another cause for aching legs, such as lumbar nerve root irritation or problems with hip, knee or poor blood supply. Treatment is directed at relieving symptoms and improving appearance. Varicose veins are incurable but the symptoms can be helped. General measures include elevating the legs, no prolonged standing or sitting, and regular exercise, including only short stretches of prolonged activities. Elastic stockings are helpful but bandages and tight socks cut off the blood flow.

Consequent dermatitis may be treated by saline or water compresses, and ulcers with zinc bandages or skin grafts. Surgery can remove the veins involved but recurrences occur. The veins can also be injected with sclerosing or hardening agents which close the vein when they become firm.

**HERBAL TREATMENT: Witch hazel** and **yarrow**, for their strong astringent and tonic properties; **calendula** as a topical ointment; **tea tree** as an astringent topical oil; **garlic**, **echinacea**, **ginseng**, **rosehip** and other herbs for their abilities to boost the circulatory system.

**OTHER USEFUL NATURAL REMEDIES:** Weight loss, gentle exercise, a high-fiber low-fat diet, avoiding alcohol and smoking, can all assist varicose veins. Supplements include vitamin C with bioflavonoids, vitamin E, cod liver oil and zinc. Sitz baths can be beneficial, as can comfrey or stinging nettle poultices. Ulcers may be helped by a combination of St. John's wort, calendula and comfrey ointments.

## Glossary

**Anodyne** An anodyne is a substance that relieves or lessens pain. It acts by removing the cause of pain, by soothing the irritated nerves of the painful part, or by desensitizing the part of the brain by which the painful impression is received.

**Antibacterial** A substance that kills or inhibits the growth or replication of bacteria.

**Antibiotic** The term used to describe any antibacterial agent derived from microorganisms, such as penicillin and streptomycin, that destroys or inhibits the growth of other microorganisms. Antibiotics are used to treat infections caused by organisms that are sensitive to them, usually bacteria or fungi.

**Anticatarrhal** An agent that helps to break down excessive secretion of thick phlegm or mucus from the mucous membranes of the nose, nasal sinuses, nasopharynx or air passages.

**Anti-inflammatory** A substance that counteracts or reduces inflammation (the reaction of the tissues to any injury, usually presenting as redness, heat, pain and swelling).

**Antioxidant** A chemical or other agent that inhibits or retards oxidation of a substance to which it is added.

**Antirheumatic** Pertaining to the relief of symptoms of any painful or immobilizing disorder of the musculoskeletal system.

**Antiseptic** A substance that tends to inhibit the growth and reproduction of disease-causing bacteria and other microorganisms. Antiseptics are used externally to cleanse wounds and internally to treat some infections.

**Antispasmodic** A drug that prevents spasms of smooth muscles, that is, muscles within the uterus, the digestive system, or the urinary tract.

**Astringent** A substance that causes contraction of tissues on application. It is usually used locally to tighten and protect the skin.

**Carminative** This term originates from the Latin word, carminare, to cleanse; today, it applies more specifically to a substance that is used for the removal of gases that have accumulated in the stomach and intestines.

**Nicholas Culpepper** Seventeenth-century apothecary, astrologer and herbalist, who first published an English translation of the *College of Physician's Pharmacopoeia*, thus making its contents available for the first time to the poor.

**Decoction** The boiling of a substance for up to an hour, then straining and standing before using at room temperature. Usually used for roots, barks, twigs and some berries. The standard quantity should be made fresh daily and drunk hot or cold.

**Demulcents** Also called "mucilaginous agents," these are soothing agents that help reduce inflammation and irritability of mucous membranes.

**Diaphoretic** Also called "sudorific" — a substance promoting profuse perspiration.

**Diuretic** A drug that promotes the formation and excretion of urine; therefore, it reduces the volume of fluid in the body.

**Diverticulitis** The inflammation of one or more diverticulain the bowel. These are pouch-like herniations, or protrusions, through the muscle layer of the large intestine, especially the lower or sigmoid intestine (or colon).

**Dysmenorrhea** Pain associated with menstruation, which can include nausea, vomiting, headache and cramps.

**Emollient** A substance that softens and soothes tissues, particularly the skin and mucous membranes.

**Extract** A substance, usually a biologically active ingredient of a plant, prepared by the use of solvents or evaporation, to separate the substance from the original material.

**Febrifuge** Synonymous with antipyretic, a substance or procedure that reduces fever.

**Fibromyalgia syndrome** A form of non-joint rheumatism characterized by musculoskeletal pain, spasm and stiffness, fatigue and severe sleep disturbance.

**John Gerard** Sixteenth-century herbalist, best known for his work *Herball or General Historie of Plantes* (1597).

**Infusion** The steeping in boiling water of a substance, such as herbs, to extract its medicinal properties — made in a similar fashion to tea. This method is usually used for the flowers and leafy parts of plants, and should be made fresh each day.

**Naturopathy** Originally a system of therapeutics based on using natural foods, light, massage, fresh air, and exercise, naturopathy now encompasses the view of treating the person as a whole, rather than just treating symptoms. It incorporates many modalities, such as herbal medicine, homeopathy, nutrition, massage and counseling. Naturopaths believe that illnesses can be healed by the natural processes of the body, with assistance from natural remedies.

**Nervine** A substance used to specifically treat the nerves of the body, usually aimed at strengthening or sedating nerve impulses and assisting in the relief of nerve conditions.

**NSAIDS** Non-steroidal anti-inflammatory drugs — any of a group of drugs having antipyretic (fever reducing), analgesic and anti-inflammatory effects. Frequently used for treatment of mild to moderate pain, the arthritic conditions, fever, non-rheumatic inflammation and dysmenorrhea.

**Palliative** Therapy which relieves or reduces the intensity of uncomfortable symptoms, but does not actually cure the disease.

**Purgative** A strong medication, usually administered by mouth, to promote emptying of the bowels.

**Tincture** Made by steeping a dried or fresh herb in a mixture of alcohol and water. The alcohol acts as a preservative, and will keep for up to two years. Only small amounts of the end product are prescribed medicinally.

**Toner** A term describing an agent that will tighten and revitalize – frequently used for skin treatments.

**Tonic** A medicinal substance that aids the general condition of the body systems to function at peak performance (such as bitters, used to promote digestion), and also to support mucous membranes, help salivary and mucous glands to secrete, and stimulate appetite.

# INDEX

## ACKNOWLEDGMENTS

For one reason or another, we'd like to thank:

Lawrie Ball, Airdre Grant, Mary-Louise Healey, Peter Keating, Cindy and Bruce Taylor, Martha Weiderman, Hans Wohlmuth Gaelon and Shannon — and the many other people (ancient and modern) who helped with this book.

## PICTURE CREDITS

### Bridgeman Art Library

page 2 – Representations of Medicinal Plants, illuminated copy of Greek Herbal of Pseudo-Apuleius, Latin, 2. 1200, British Library, London/Bridgeman Art Library, London/New York

page 7 – Administering Medicinal Herbs, 1534 (woodcut) by Polish School (16th century), Philadelphia Museum of Art/Bridgeman Art Library, London/New York

page 15 – Medicago sativa (Alfalfa), plate 2111, illustration from "Icones Florae Germanicae Helveticae ...", engraved by Scherell by German School (19th century), Natural History Museum, London/Bridgeman Art Library, London/New York

page 35 – Allium sativum, published by Dr. Woodville, 1792. L'Acquaforte, London/Bridgeman Art Library, London/New York

page 37 – Gentianaceae (the Gentian tribe), from "Illustrations of the Natural Orders of Plants" by Elizabeth Twining (1805–89), British Library, London/Bridgeman Art Library, London/New York

page 39 – Ginger, 1988 by Julie Virtue (living artist), Private Collection/Bridgeman Art Library, London/New York

page 43 – Ginseng, Bridgeman Art Library

page 45 – Horse Chestnut, Bridgeman Art Library

page 47 – Licorice, Bridgeman Art Library

page 49 – Marshmallow, Bridgeman Art Library

page 59 – Raspberry, Bridgeman Art Library

page 73 – Thyme, Bridgeman Art Library

page 79 – Witchhazel, Bridgeman Art Library

### et archive

Cover – Dandelion from Jean Bourdichon Hours of Anne of Burgundy, Bibliotheque Nationale Paris/e.t. archive

page 51 – Meadowsweet, e.t. archive

page 63 – Rosemary

page 83 – 15th century merchant selling herb thyme, Biblioteca Estense Moderia/e.t. archive

### Ivy Hansen

15, 17, 21, 29, 30, 33, 45, 18, 48, 54, 59, 63, 71 74, 81

# DISCLAIMER

This book is intended to give general information only and is not a substitute for professional and medical advice. Consult your health care provider before adopting any of the treatments contained in this book. The publisher, author and distributor expressly disclaim all liability to any person arising directly or indirectly from the use of, or for any errors or omissions in, the information in this book. The adoption and application of the information in this book is at the reader's discretion and is their sole responsibility.

This edition published in 1999 by SMITHMARK Publishers, a division of U.S. Media Holdings, Inc., 115 West 18th Street, New York, NY 10011

SMITHMARK books are available for bulk purchase for sales promotion and premium use. For details write or call the manager of special sales, SMITHMARK Publishers 115 West 18th Street, New York, NY 10011

Produced by Lansdowne Publishing Pty Ltd, Sydney First published in 1999

Kerr, Gillian N.D.
        Modern ailments. ancient remedies : healing manual / Gillian Kerr and Yvonnne Bloomfield.
        p.    cm.
        ISBN 0-7651-1681-2 (hardcover)
        1. Herbs--Therapeutic use--Handbooks. manuals, etc. 2. Materia medica, Vegetable--Handbooks, manuals, etc. 3. Traditional medicine--Handbooks, manuals, etc. I. Bloomfield, Yvonne. II. Title.
        RM666. H33K456  1999
        615'.321--dc21                                                    99-17080

Set in Janson Text on QuarkXPress
Printed in Singapore by Tien Wah Press (Pte) Ltd

10  9  8  7  6  5  4  3  2  1

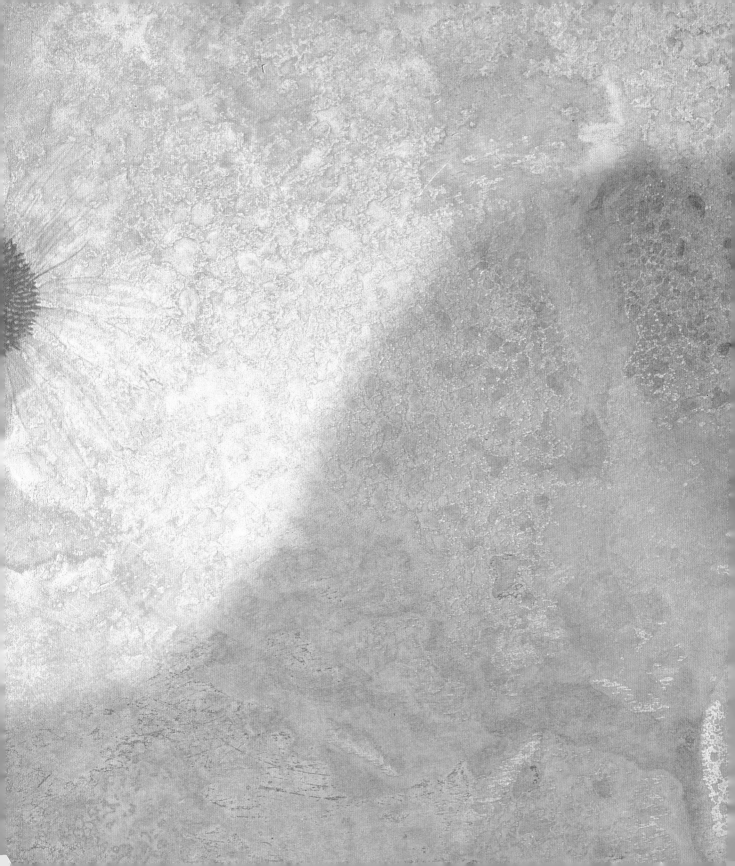